T0221513

FRACTURES OF THE SHOULDER GIRDLE

EDITED BY

WILLIAM N. LEVINE
LOUIS U. BIGLIANI
*Columbia University, College of Physicians and Surgeons
and New York-Presbyterian Hospital
New York, New York, U.S.A.*

GUIDO MARRA
*Loyola University Medical Center
Maywood, Illinois, U.S.A.*

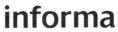

healthcare

New York   London

Informa Healthcare USA, Inc.
52 Vanderbilt Avenue
New York, NY 10017

© 2009 by Informa Healthcare USA, Inc. (original copyright 2003 by Marcel Dekker, Inc.)
Informa Healthcare is an Informa business

No claim to original U.S. Government works
Printed in the United States of America on acid-free paper
10 9 8 7 6 5 4 3 2

International Standard Book Number-10: 0-8247-0898-9 (Hardcover)
International Standard Book Number-13: 978-0-8247-0898-6 (Hardcover)

Visit the Informa Web site at
www.informa.com

and the Informa Healthcare Web site at
www.informahealthcare.com

To my wife Jill and my daughter Sonya Belle Levine.
W. N. L.

To my wife Katherine, my children, and my family for their love and support.
G. M.

To my wife Annie and my daughters Anne-Louise and Suzie.
L. U. B.

Preface

Treatment of shoulder girdle fractures remains one of the most challenging problems in orthopedic surgery. The complex anatomy of the shoulder intertwined with the intricate motion of the shoulder has led to frustrating results with nonoperative and operative treatments alike. This book offers explanations for some of these complexities and provides up-to-date approaches from some of the world's leaders in shoulder and upper extremity surgery.

Classification of proximal humeral fractures is elegantly introduced in the first chapter. Chapter 2 shares a wealth of experience with percutaneous treatment of proximal humeral fractures. Open reduction and internal fixation with a variety of implant choices are covered in Chapters 3–6. Chapter 7 gives a beautifully illustrated description of humeral head replacement for displaced four-part proximal humeral fractures. Next, Chapter 8 presents the authors' experience with arthroscopic treatment of proximal humeral fractures. Chapter 9 provides practical and up-to-date advice on the management of difficult nonunions of the clavicle and the proximal humerus. Chapters 10–13 deal with some of the more complex problems involving the shoulder girdle, including malunions, locked dislocations, scapula and glenoid fractures, and clavicle malunions. Last, Chapter 14 provides a thorough review of surgical approaches to the humeral shaft. It is our hope that this book will serve as a "how-to" guide when orthopedic surgeons are faced with the treatment of fractures of the shoulder girdle.

We would like to thank all those—family, friends, and mentors—who have been instrumental in making this book possible.

William N. Levine
Guido Marra
Louis U. Bigliani

Contents

Contributors

Carl J. Basamania, M.D. Assistant Professor, Division of Orthopaedic Surgery, Department of Surgery, Duke University Medical Center, and Chief, Durham Veterans Administration Hospital, Durham, North Carolina, U.S.A.

Gregory S. Bauer, M.D. Goldsboro Orthopaedic Associates, Goldsboro, North Carolina, U.S.A.

Louis U. Bigliani, M.D. Frank E. Stinchfield Professor and Chairman, Department of Orthopedic Surgery, Columbia University, College of Physicians and Surgeons, New York-Presbyterian Hospital, and Director, Center for Shoulder, Elbow and Sports Medicine, New York, New York, U.S.A.

Theodore A. Blaine, M.D. Assistant Professor, Department of Orthopaedic Surgery, Columbia University, College of Physicians and Surgeons, New York-Presbyterian Hospital, Associate Director, Center for Shoulder, Elbow and Sports Medicine, and New York-Presbyterian Hospital, New York, New York, U.S.A.

Sergio L. Checchia, Prof.Dr. Chief, Shoulder and Elbow Group, Department of Orthopedics, Santa Casa Hospitals and School of Medicine, São Paulo, Brazil

Evan L. Flatow, M.D. Lasker Professor, Department of Orthopaedic Surgery, Mount Sinai School of Medicine, and Chief, Division of Shoulder Surgery, Department of Surgery, Mount Sinai Medical Center, New York, New York, U.S.A.

Michael Q. Freehill, M.D. Assistant Professor, Department of Orthopaedic Surgery, University of Minnesota, Minneapolis, Minnesota, U.S.A.

Leesa M. Galatz, M.D. Assistant Professor, Shoulder and Elbow Service, Department of Orthopaedic Surgery, Washington University School of Medicine, and Barnes-Jewish Hospital, St. Louis, Missouri, U.S.A.

Ariane Gerber, M.D. Chief, Upper Extremity Unit, Department of Trauma and Reconstructive Surgery, Campus Virchow-Klinikum, Humboldt University, Berlin, Germany

David L. Glaser, M.D. The Cali Family Assistant Professor of Orthopaedic Surgery and Associate Professor, University of Pennsylvania Shoulder and Elbow Service, University of Pennsylvania and Hospital of the University of Pennsylvania, Philadelphia, Pennsylvania, U.S.A.

Yassamin Hazrati, M.D. Department of Orthopaedic Surgery, Kaiser Permanente Medical Center, Vallejo, California, U.S.A.

Clemens Hübner, M.D. Department of Traumatology, General Hospital Salzburg, Salzburg, Austria

Christopher K. Jones, M.D. Southern Orthopaedics/Sports Medicine, La Grange, Georgia, U.S.A.

Jesse B. Jupiter, M.D. Professor, Department of Orthopaedic Surgery, Harvard Medical School, and Chief, Division of Hand Surgery, Department of Orthopaedic Surgery, Massachusetts General Hospital, Boston, Massachusetts, U.S.A.

Steven J. Klepps, M.D. Orthopedic Associates, Yellowstone Medical Center, Billings, Montana, U.S.A.

William N. Levine, M.D. Assistant Professor, Department of Orthopaedic Surgery, Columbia University, College of Physicians and Surgeons, New York-Presbyterian Hospital, and Associate Director, Center for Shoulder, Elbow and Sports Medicine, New York, New York, U.S.A.

Guido Marra, M.D. Director, Shoulder and Elbow Surgery, and Assistant Professor, Department of Orthopaedic Surgery, Loyola University Medical Center, Maywood, Illinois, U.S.A.

Anand M. Murthi, M.D. Assistant Professor, Shoulder and Elbow Service, Department of Orthopaedics, University of Maryland School of Medicine, Baltimore, Maryland, U.S.A.

Matthew L. Ramsey, M.D. Assistant Professor, Department of Orthopaedic Surgery, University of Pennsylvania School of Medicine, and Hospital of the University of Pennsylvania, Philadelphia, Pennsylvania, U.S.A.

Herbert Resch, M.D. Head, Department of Traumatology, General Hospital Salzburg, Salzburg, Austria

David Ring, M.D. Instructor, Department of Orthopaedic Surgery, Harvard Medical School, and Hand and Upper Extremity Service, Department of Orthopaedic Surgery, Massachusetts General Hospital, Boston, Massachusetts, U.S.A.

Andreas M. Sauerbrey, M.D. Orthopaedics of Steamboat Springs, Steamboat Springs, Colorado, U.S.A.

Felix H. Savoie III, M.D. Codirector, Upper Extremity Services, Mississippi Sports Medicine and Orthopaedic Center, Jackson, Mississippi, U.S.A.

Michael D. Stover, M.D. Assistant Professor, Department of Orthopaedic Surgery, Loyola University Medical Center, Maywood, Illinois, U.S.A.

Jon J. P. Warner, M.D. Chief, Harvard Shoulder Service, Partners Department of Orthopaedics, Massachusetts General Hospital and Brigham & Women's Hospital, Boston, Massachusetts, U.S.A.

Gerald R. Williams, Jr., M.D. Chief, Shoulder and Elbow Service, Department of Orthopaedic Surgery, University of Pennsylvania School of Medicine, Philadelphia, Pennsylvania, U.S.A.

Ken Yamaguchi, M.D. Associate Professor and Chief, Shoulder and Elbow Service, Department of Orthopaedic Surgery, Washington University School of Medicine, and Barnes-Jewish Hospital, St. Louis, Missouri, U.S.A.

1

Classification of Proximal Humerus Fractures

STEVEN J. KLEPPS

Yellowstone Medical Center, Billings, Montana, U.S.A.

YASSAMIN HAZRATI

Kaiser Permanente Medical Center, Vallejo, California, U.S.A.

EVAN L. FLATOW

Mount Sinai School of Medicine and Mount Sinai Medical Center, New York, New York, U.S.A.

I INTRODUCTION

Fractures of the proximal humerus are relatively common, accounting for 2–4% of upper extremity fractures (29), with 75% occurring after age 60 and a 3:1 female-to-male incidence. Most proximal humeral fractures (over 85%) are nondisplaced and amenable to nonoperative measures. The therapeutic challenge lies in the remaining 15% of displaced fractures, which can vary widely in comminution, bone quality, and fracture location (4,44). The advent or at least popularization of percutaneous techniques has certainly modified the surgical indications for proximal humerus fractures and has recently spurred debate on the proper treatment of these injuries (1,3,30,68). In the end, however, the selection of proper surgical candidates and fixation techniques depends upon the accurate assessment of these fractures.

At least some of the controversy as to the optimal fixation method is due to inconsistent or inaccurate fracture classification. This may result from ambiguities in the classification system employed, inadequate observer experience, and reliance on sub-optimal radiographs. The proximal humerus is a particularly difficult structure to image, since the scapula floats on the chest wall and the humerus can rotate freely on the glenoid. Slight changes in beam orientation can dramatically shift apparent bone relationships (Fig. 1). The use of computed tomography (CT) scans or magnetic resonance imaging (MRI) as a substitute for personally repositioning the patient to obtain adequate radiographs may actually further confuse the picture (Fig. 2) (2,62).

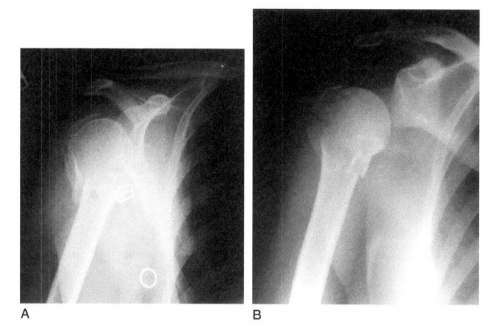

A   B

Figure 1 Effect of radiographic position on fracture evaluation. (A) The AP radiograph of the proximal humerus fracture in internal rotation shows a nondisplaced surgical neck fracture with a displaced greater tuberosity fracture. (B) The scapular AP radiograph in external rotation as positioned by the orthopedic surgeon shows a minimally displaced greater tuberosity fracture in profile.

Appropriate treatment of proximal humerus fractures, then, depends on an understanding of anatomy, accurate imaging techniques, and proper classification of the fracture type.

II ANATOMY

Before describing the classification of proximal humerus fractures, it is important to have a thorough understanding of the bony landmarks, the position of the muscular anatomy, the relevant neurovascular structures, and, most importantly, the rotator cuff muscles.

A Humerus

The humeral shaft connects with the proximal portion at the surgical neck, just below the greater and lesser tuberosities at the metaphyseal flare. The anatomical neck is above the tuberosities, between the articular margin of the head and the attachment of the articular capsule. The most common site of fracture is the surgical neck, while fractures at the anatomical neck are exceedingly rare. The greater tuberosity is much more commonly fractured than the lesser tuberosity. The final site of fracture is the articular surface, which results in head-splitting or chondral fractures.

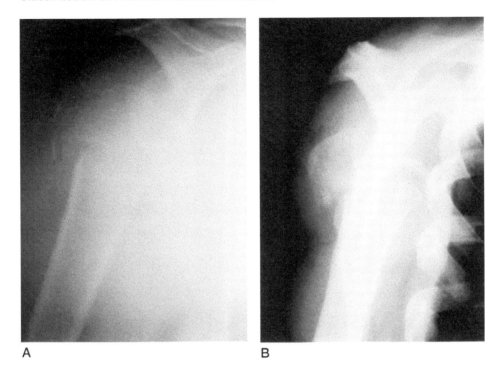

A   B

Figure 2 Head-splitting fracture of the proximal humerus. In the original AP view in internal rotation (A) and Y-lateral view (B), the fracture is not well visualized, and therefore a CT scan was obtained (C). This did not show the fracture well as the fracture line was in parallel with the beam of the CT, but the scout view (D) did show a displaced head-splitting fracture further confirmed on an AP view in better orientation (E).

The proximal humeral articular surface is a segment of a sphere with a diameter ranging from 37 to 57 mm (7). The head is inclined an average of 130 degrees to the shaft. The geometric center of the head is offset an average of 3 mm posteriorly and 7 mm medially from the center of the shaft. The subchondral bone is fairly strong, but the density of the humeral neck and the cancellous bone inside the proximal humerus decreases with age (24,57,58). Humeral retroversion has been reported to range between 18 and 40 degrees (7,11,27,38,40,47,51,52) with a side-to-side difference often noted (7,11). The large range of values found throughout these studies has led to a recent trend in restoring the preexisting anatomy using consistent landmarks such as the biceps groove or cuff insertion (66). However, if the local anatomy is shattered, the process becomes more difficult, especially when performing humeral replacement.

B Proximal Humerus Muscles

The most significant muscle for shaft displacement is the pectoralis major, which pulls the humeral shaft anteriorly and medially (Fig. 3). The rotator cuff muscles most significantly affect the tuberosities and head rotation.

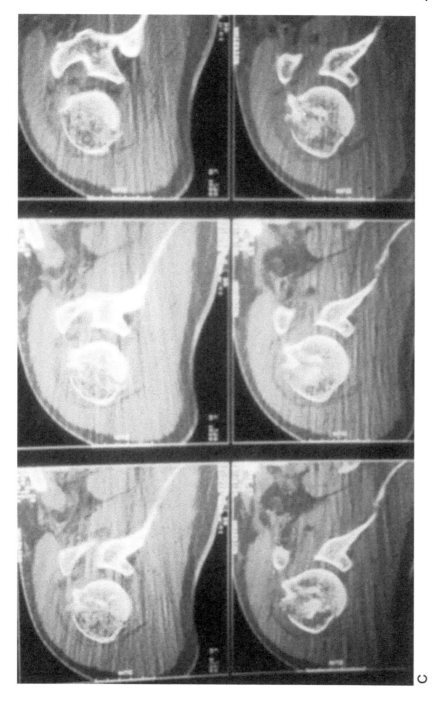

Figure 2 Continued

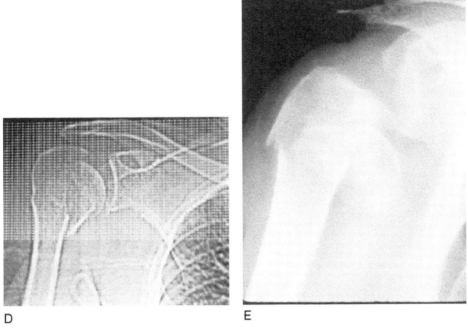

D   E

Figure 2 Continued

The greater tuberosity has three facets for insertion of the tendons of the supraspinatus, infraspinatus, and teres minor muscles. These facets can fracture separately or as a whole. The tendon of the subscapularis inserts on the lesser tuberosity. The bicipital groove, bridged by the transverse humeral ligament and containing the long head of the biceps, runs between the tuberosities. Associated rotator cuff tears are rare, and, therefore, the tuberosities are generally retracted in the direction of the intact rotator cuff (Fig. 3). Greater tuberosity fractures may retract posteriorly and superiorly by the pull of the supraspinatus and infraspinatus. In isolated lesser tuberosity fractures, the subscapularis pulls the fragment medially. At other times, an intact rotator interval between the supraspinatus and subscapularis may limit displacement of isolated greater tuberosity fractures.

For surgical neck fractures associated with lesser tuberosity fractures and intact greater tuberosities (three-part lesser tuberosity fractures), external rotation of the humeral head takes place. For three-part greater tuberosity fractures where the lesser tuberosity remains intact, on the other hand, the head is rotated internally. Neer referred to this spinning of the head in three-part fractures as "rotatory subluxation."

C Vascular Anatomy

Classification schemes are useful when they are effective in both predicting prognosis and determining treatment. The association between fracture location and vascular

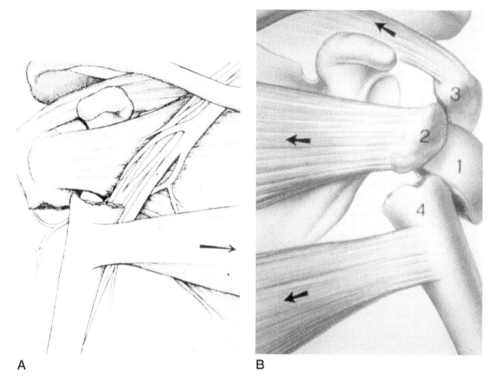

A   B

Figure 3 Muscular anatomy associated with proximal humerus fractures. (A) A surgical neck fracture is shown exemplifying the anterior and medial pull of the pectoralis major on the humeral shaft. (B) A four-part proximal humerus fracture with the dislocated head devoid of soft tissue (1). The deformity caused by the various attached muscles is shown with the subscapularis pulling the lesser tuberosity anteriorly and medially (2), the supraspinatus and infraspinatus pulling the greater tuberosity superiorly and posteriorly (3), and the pectoralis major again pulling the humeral shaft anteriorly and medially (4).

anatomy plays a role in determining patient outcome and, thus, is important to understand when classifying these injuries. The important vessels to consider are the axillary artery and its distal branches, the anterior and posterior humeral circumflex vessels. The anterior humeral circumflex artery gives rise to the arcuate artery (artery of Laing) and continues laterally around the shaft to anastamose with the posterior humeral circumflex artery. Because of the close adherence and proximity of these vessels, vascular injuries can occur from four-part fracture/dislocations or well-meaning attempts at their reduction. Axillary artery injury most commonly occurs at the origin of these circumflex vessels (Fig. 4).

The main arterial supply to the humeral head arises from the anterior humeral circumflex artery (17,21,41,45,56). Its anterolateral branch enters the head to form the arcuate artery and supplies all but a small posterior part of the head (21). Many extraosseous collaterals can help feed the arcuate artery if the anterior humeral circumflex vessels are ligated proximal to these anastamoses. However, if the blood supply is interrupted close to the entry of the anterolateral branch into bone, the

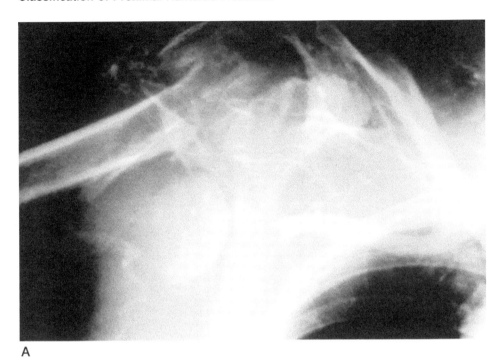

A

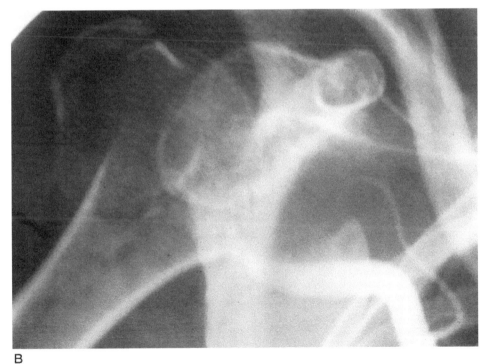

B

Figure 4 Angiograms of proximal humerus fractures resulting in vascular injury. (A) The axillary artery is tamponaded by the humeral head resting in the axilla. (B) A spike on the proximal humeral shaft obstructs the axillary artery.

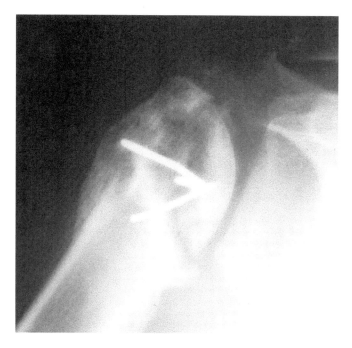

Figure 5 Previous proximal humerus fracture that underwent open reduction and internal fixation resulted in avascular necrosis of the humeral head.

blood supply to the head might be compromised (21). Recent studies have found that the humeral head can still be perfused despite complete ligation of the anterolateral branch just before it penetrated the head (8). Therefore, it may be a combination of injury and extensive soft tissue stripping from either the associated dislocation or operative exposure that has led to the increased incidence of avascular necrosis in four-part fracture/dislocations (Fig. 5) (6,14,16,20,23,33,37,43,53,64,65).

D   Nerves

A complete neurovascular examination of the upper extremity is essential, especially in complex fractures or dislocations, as axillary artery and brachial plexus injuries have been reported with increasing frequency in these injuries (26,69). The axillary nerve is most often injured, as it lies on the deep surface of the deltoid and wraps around the proximal humerus before traversing the quadrilateral space. It divides into three major branches that supply motor innervation to the teres minor and deltoid muscles. The lateral brachial cutaneous nerve penetrates the deltoid to provide sensation to the overlying skin.

The shoulder is innervated primarily by the brachial plexus (C5-T1) with contributions from the C3 and C4 nerves. Above the clavicle the roots coalesce to form the upper (C5, C6), middle (C7), and lower (C7, T1) trunks. The lateral, posterior, and medial cords arise below the clavicle, their names reflecting their position relative to the axillary artery. The axillary nerve and subscapular nerves originate from the posterior cord with the axillary providing innervation for the deltoid and teres minor, while the upper and lower subscapular nerves provide innervation for the subscapularis. The suprascapular nerve, which originates from the upper trunk, innervates the supraspinatus and infraspinatus. The articular branches to the shoulder joint arise primarily from the axillary, suprascapular, and lateral anterior thoracic nerves (19). The sympathetic ganglion and posterior cord also supply occasional branches.

III PATHOMECHANICS OF THE PROXIMAL HUMERAL FRACTURE

Most proximal humeral fractures occur in elderly patients with osteoporotic bone (28); however, significant trauma can lead to this injury at any age. The fracture can be caused by direct blow to the upper arm (34,35,42) or by indirect violence such as humeral contact with the acromion or glenoid rim. In addition, traction from the rotator cuff tendons can avulse the tuberosities (9,22). The decreased incidence of isolated greater tuberosity fractures in elderly patients may represent age-related weakening of the rotator cuff tendons and their decreased contribution to an avulsion force (28). Another proposed mechanism is a strong muscular contraction such as in the setting of electric shock or seizure, which, of course, is rare (32,59). Attempts to use the mechanism of injury to classify proximal humerus fractures have been made in the past, but fracture location and displacement have been found more useful.

It is, in fact, the muscle forces rather than the mechanism of injury that contribute to fragment displacement (Fig. 3). The shaft is generally drawn anteromedially by the force of the pectoralis major (18). The greater tuberosity is drawn posteriorly by the infraspinatus and teres minor and superiorly by the supraspinatus (15,49,50). The subscapularis places medial and internal rotational forces on the fragments to which it remains attached.

IV DIAGNOSIS

Proximal humeral fractures occur in all segments of the population. Older patients tend to have isolated fractures, while younger patients are more likely to sustain associated injuries due to the higher amount of energy involved (55). Therefore, the entire upper extremity should be palpated for evidence of other injuries. Rib fractures have also been reported in association with proximal humeral fractures (25). Important considerations include the mechanism of injury and the amount of energy required to sustain the injury.

The signs and symptoms of proximal humeral fractures are typical of most fractures. Pain is present with any attempt at motion or palpation. Inspection reveals swelling and ecchymosis, which appears 24–48 hours after injury and may extend distally into the arm, forearm, chest wall, or breast for the next 4–5 days. Crepitus can be noted with motion of the fracture fragments. Fracture stability can be assessed by gently rotating the humeral shaft while palpating the proximal portion of the humerus. The fracture is stable if the pieces move as a unit, which can be useful in classifying these injuries.

A complete neurovascular exam should be performed as isolated axillary nerve and mixed brachial plexus injuries are the most common neurological injuries found after proximal humeral fractures (4,63). The finding of asymmetrical radial pulses may be a subtle clue to arterial injuries, and an angiogram should be performed. Arterial injury should be suspected in all four-part fracture/dislocations in which the head segment is in the axilla, even in the absence of vascular findings (Fig. 4). It is useful when performing surgery in such cases to have a vascular team available, and to exercise great caution in removing the head from the axilla, as it may have tamponaded an arterial injury or be adherent to the arterial wall.

V IMAGING

Careful, accurate radiographs are necessary and usually sufficient to determine the extent of injury and subsequently classify the proximal humeral fractures. The treating surgeon must be sure that adequate films are obtained, personally positioning the patient if necessary. The "trauma series" consists of an anterior-posterior (true AP) scapular view, a lateral "Y-view" of the scapula, and an axillary view of the glenohumeral joint (Fig. 6). The Velpeau axillary view is preferred for acute fractures since the arm remains in the sling (Fig. 6) (5). If the fracture is stable, the surgeon may elect to place the arm in slight external rotation for the scapular AP view to place the greater tuberosity in profile (Fig. 1).

Although plain radiographs are usually sufficient, CT scans and MRIs can occasionally be helpful. CT scans can be used to glean additional data such as glenoid fractures, posterior dislocations, and posteriorly displaced greater tuberosity

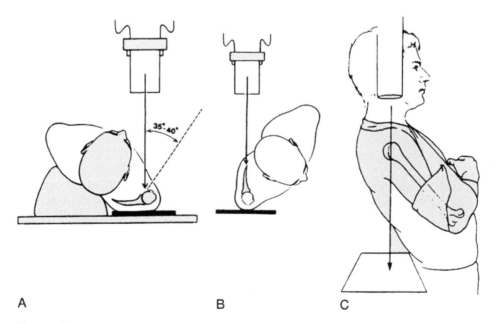

A   B   C

Figure 6   Radiographic trauma series: (A) true scapular AP radiograph; (B) Y-lateral view of the scapula; (C) Velpeau axillary view. (From Ref. 70.)

or medially displaced lesser tuberosity fragments (Fig. 7). MRIs are not used routinely, but can be helpful in diagnosing nondisplaced fractures (Fig. 8).

A fractured greater tuberosity fragment may remain as one piece or become comminuted, resulting in the facets separating along the pull of their respective muscles. It is important to recognize this and not, for example, repair the obviously superiorly displaced supraspinatus facet down while leaving the infraspinatus facet posteriorly and medially retracted. These facets can often be seen radiographically but may occasionally require operative evaluation.

VI PROXIMAL HUMERAL FRACTURE CLASSIFICATION

A classification system for proximal humerus fractures should provide a comprehensive means of describing all relevant fracture fragments and dislocations. This, in turn, should aid in determining treatment and long-term prognosis. As with any classification system it should have an acceptable level of inter- and intraobserver reliability necessary for comparison of different treatment methods. Finally, the classification should be based on a standard, easily obtained radiographic series. Although often criticized, the Neer classification for proximal humeral fractures remains the standard system and is the focus of our discussion. To better understand the Neer classification, we will review both its historical origins and recent studies evaluating its reliability. Finally, we will detail the original description through radiographic examples.

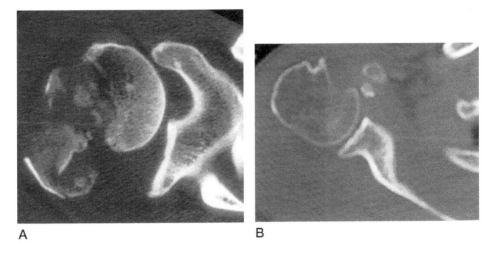

A   B

Figure 7 CT scans of tuberosity fractures can be helpful in determining the extent of tuberosity displacement. (A) This widely displaced greater tuberosity fragment was also visible on plain radiographs, making this CT unhelpful in treatment decisions. (B) This lesser tuberosity fracture was less well visualized on plain radiographs; the CT showed the true amount of displacement.

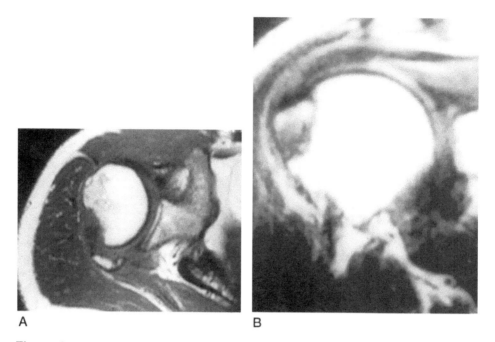

A   B

Figure 8 MRI of two separate greater tuberosity fractures exemplifying the role of MRI. (A) This posteriorly displaced greater tuberosity fragment was also evident on plain radiographs. (B) This nondisplaced greater tuberosity fracture was not evident on plain radiographs while clearly shown on this MRI.

A   Historical Development

Original fracture classifications focused on the location of the fracture, but did not account for multiple fracture lines or dislocations. Kocher first divided proximal humerus fractures into supratubercular, pertubercular, infratubercular, and subtubercular (36). Codman more accurately described but did not classify the fractures as occurring along the lines of the epiphyseal scars and noted four possible fragments: the articular surface, humeral shaft, greater tuberosity, and lesser tuberosity (Fig. 9) (9).

Subsequent classification schemes focused on mechanism of injury such as the Watson-Jones' classification, which described impacted adduction, impacted abduction, and a minimally displaced "contusion-crack" fracture (67). The abduction and adduction fractures can be confused, however, if the humerus rotation is changed during radiography (Fig. 10). Dehne felt that forced abduction separated the head, greater tuberosity, and shaft from one another, leading to a "three-fragment fracture." Forced extension, on the other hand, separated the surgical neck from the shaft into a "two-fragment fracture," while the "head-splitting fracture" resulted from the head being driven into the glenoid (12). Dehne

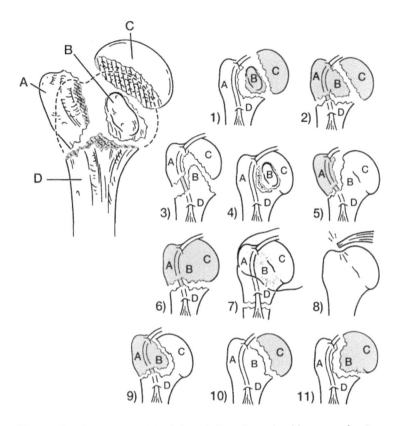

Figure 9 Codman's original description of proximal humerus fractures.

did not include lesser tuberosity fractures in his classification, although he noted the presence of more serious fractures and fracture dislocations.

Based on these previous studies (especially Codman's), Neer noticed that the degree of fracture displacement differentiated proximal humerus fracture behavior (48). He was also concerned with fracture dislocations because the head was devoid of soft tissue attachments and, therefore, susceptible to avascular necrosis. De Anquin and De Anquin employed a classification similar to Neer's in 1950 based on the division of the proximal humerus into three zones and fracture fragments (10). They had also noted a difference between impacted and nonimpacted four-part fractures. Depalma differentiated between fracture dislocations with complete loss of articular contact and rotational deformities (where the head remained in the joint capsule despite being spun) (13). Later, Neer published his classification system based on the results of his observation of 300 randomly selected displaced proximal humerus fractures (Fig. 11) (49). He emphasized the patterns of displacement rather than location of fracture lines and also focused on assessing head viability and its relationship to the glenoid.

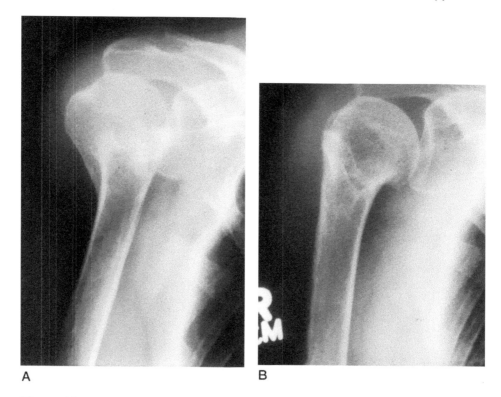

A   B

Figure 10   Radiographs of this proximal humerus fracture show an apparent mechanism of "adducted impaction" resulting in a valgus postion (A). (B) The supposed mechanism of "abducted impaction" resulting in a varus position. Both are actually radiographs of the same fracture shown in different positions of rotation.

Jakob and colleagues proposed a complex and complete fracture classification scheme that has been incorporated into the AO/ASIF classification (Fig. 12) (31,46). The AO system places more emphasis on the vascular supply of the articular portion of the proximal humerus. If either tuberosity and its associated rotator cuff remains attached to the articular segment, the vascular supply is considered adequate. One subgroup of type C fractures with valgus impaction of the head segment has received much attention because of the lower incidence of avascular necrosis. The lower rate of avascular necrosis in the valgus-impacted four-part fracture is postulated to be due to an intact medial soft tissue hinge at the anatomical neck (31,54). This allows the tuberosities to return to their anatomical positions after percutaneous elevation of the humeral head. In evaluating this AO/ASIF system for reliability, inter- and intraobserver levels even among its creators were similar to the reliability reported using Neer's system (61). The system is not commonly used today because of its multiple subgroups and general complexity. There are no long-term results of treatments using the AO/ASIF classification system.

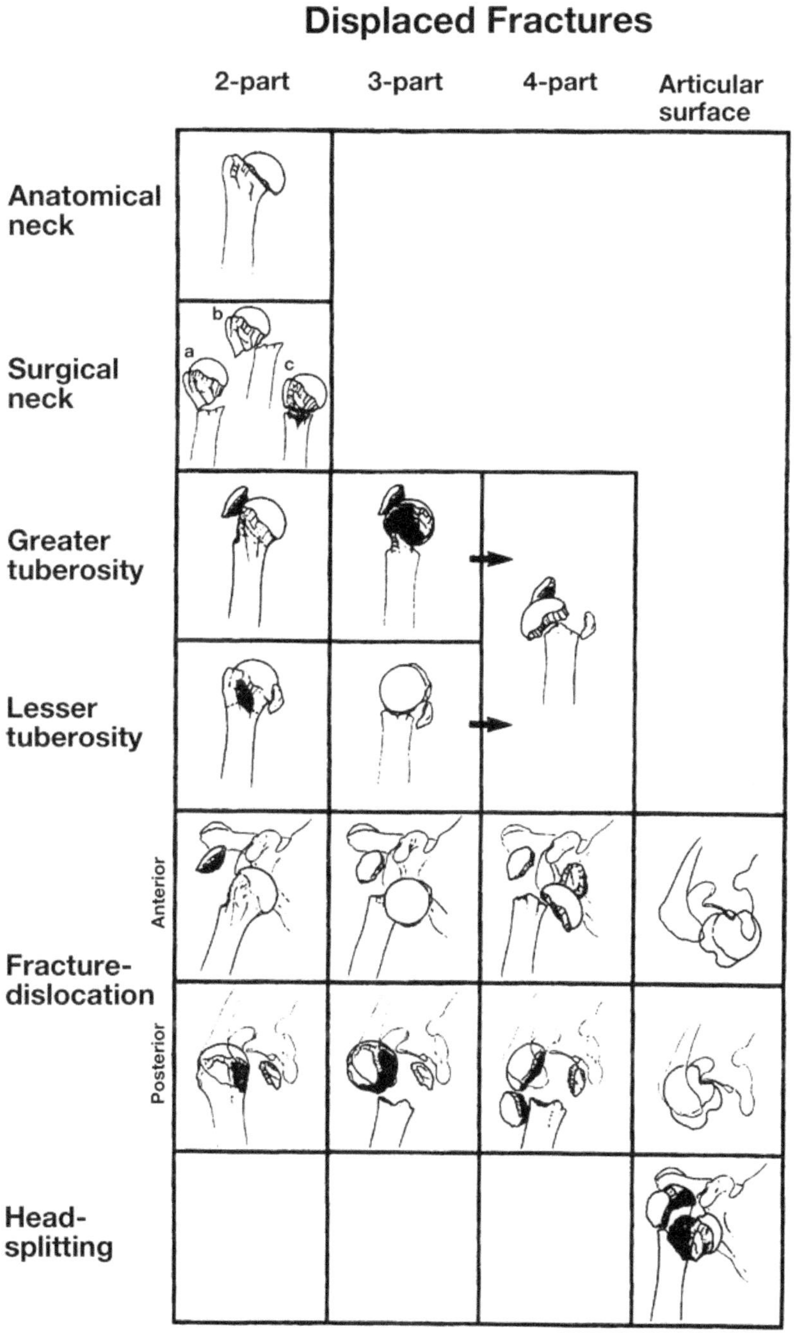

Figure 11   Neer classification of proximal humerus fractures. (From Ref. 70.)

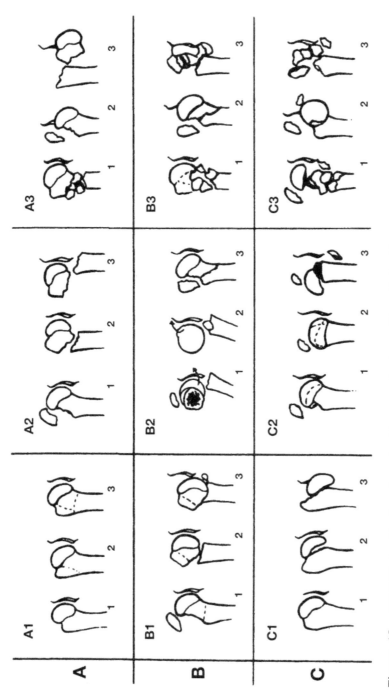

Figure 12 AO/ASIF classification of proximal humerus fractures. (From Ref. 71.)

B   Reliability of the Neer Classification

The Neer classification is by far the most widely used system for assessing proximal humeral fractures. There are several studies in the literature on its inter- and intraobserver reliability.

Kristiansen et al. found poor intraobserver reliability, especially among inexperienced observers (39). Classification was based on only AP and lateral radiographs rather than a complete trauma series. Interobserver reproducibility was not measured and a condensed version of the classification was used. Sidor et al. showed a reliability coefficient of 0.5 (moderate) for their evaluation of 50 fractures by observers of different experience levels (60). Intraobserver reliability was highest for the shoulder specialist at 0.83, "almost perfect," and lowest for the skeletal radiologist at 0.5. Siebenrock and Gerber found a mean kappa value of 0.4 (poor) and 0.6 (fair) for interobserver and intraobserver reliability, respectively, using the Neer system (61). The main difficulties were in assessing the lesser tuberosity fracture and determining the amount of fracture fragment displacement.

The effect of computed tomography on increasing reliability and reproducibility was subsequently assessed (2,62). The mean kappa coefficient for intraobserver reliability increased with CT scans in these studies, but, the interobserver reliability was unchanged.

It is helpful to remember that reliability is only one measure of the usefulness of a classification. For example, simply determining whether a fracture is open or closed would, of course, have excellent reliability. However, grading the soft tissue injury in open fractures may improve clinical decision making but reduce kappa values. Thus, a scheme with more groupings may be less reliable but more prognostic. Furthermore, imperfect reliability of a classification does not disprove the conclusions of properly performed studies using the classification system.

The statistical tests are designed to take the imprecision of the classification systems into consideration. For example, if 75% of four-part fractures develop AVN in a series and this is a statistically significantly higher rate than two-part fractures, then this conclusion remains valid whether the authors classified four-part fractures correctly 100% of the time and 75% of them developed AVN or they classified them correctly only 75% of the time but all "true" four-part fractures developed AVN. Finally, even poor-to-moderate reliability is better than rolling dice (K-value = 0) or vague descriptions such as "complex" fractures, and no classification has been shown to be more reliable than Neer's.

C   The Neer Classification System

The Neer system classifies fractures by displacement of any of the four principal fragments: humeral head, humeral shaft, greater tuberosity, and lesser tuberosity. Fragments (parts) are only considered displaced if separated by more than 1 cm (5 mm in greater tuberosity fragments) or angulated 45 degrees (Fig. 11). If no segment is displaced more than 1 cm or rotated more than 45 degrees, then the fracture is considered a one-part or nondisplaced fracture regardless of the number or location of fracture lines (Figs. 1 and 10). Two-, three-, and four-part fractures have displaced fragments.

A two-part fracture has a single displaced fragment. The most common two-part fractures are the surgical neck fractures in which the shaft is separated from the head and both attached tuberosities (Fig. 13) and greater tuberosity fractures (Figs. 14–16). Lesser tuberosity two-part fractures (Fig. 17) are rare, and anatomic neck fractures (Fig. 18) are almost never seen in isolation.

Three-part fractures are more commonly characterized by a surgical neck fracture associated with a displaced greater tuberosity fragment in which the lesser tuberosity is still attached to the articular surface (Fig. 19). Less commonly, the surgical neck fracture is associated with a displaced lesser tuberosity fragment, with the greater tuberosity still attached to the articular surface (Fig. 20).

In four-part fractures the articular surface is separated from all the other fragments, even if the tuberosities remain together. Thus, a four-part fracture can

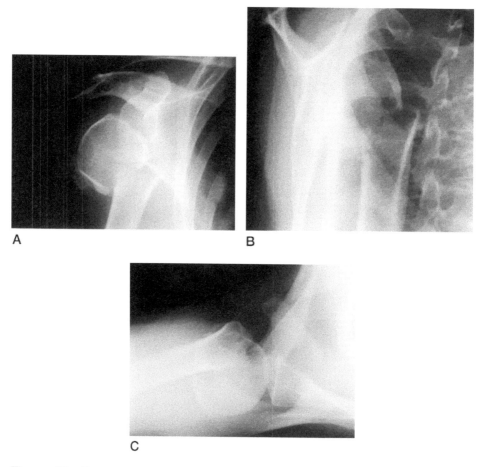

Figure 13 Two-part surgical neck fracture. (A) AP view and (B) Y-lateral view, showing the head angulated at 90°, exceeding the 45° necessary to be considered apart by Neer. (C) Axillary view shows the humeral head completely displaced from the humeral shaft.

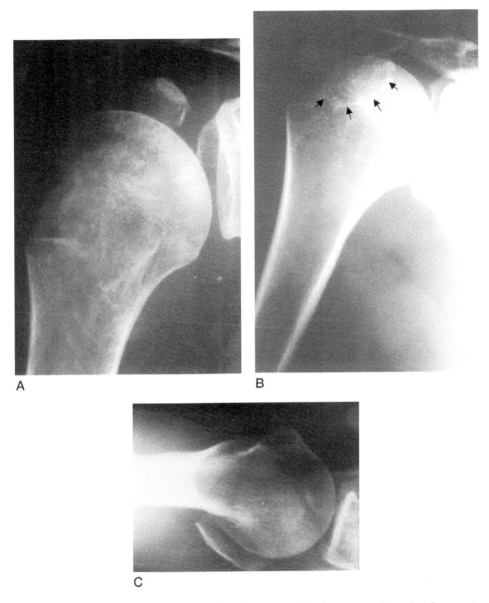

Figure 14 Two-part greater tuberosity fractures. AP views can show the fragment superiorly displaced (A) or transposed behind the humeral head (B). Therefore, it is important to take an axillary (C) view to better visualize the extent of tuberosity displacement.

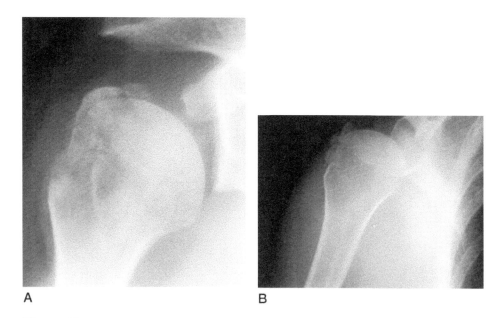

A   B

Figure 15   Two-part greater tuberosity fractures can appear as calcifications as shown in these two greater tuberosity fractures.

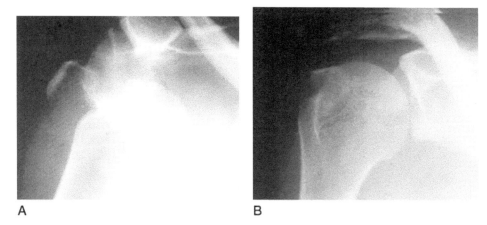

A   B

Figure 16   Two-part greater tuberosity fractures can be associated with anterior dislocations (A). After closed reduction, the tuberosity in this fracture reduced (B) and did not require surgery. Therefore, the fracture should be classified after reduction when determining a treatment plan.

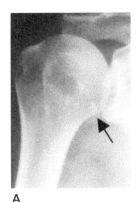

A

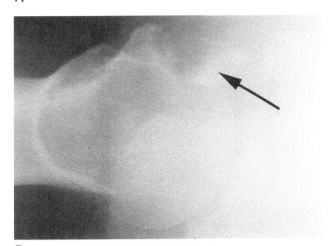

B

C

Figure 17 Two-part lesser tuberosity fracture. Less common variant with the lesser tuberosity pulled medially, as seen in the AP view (A) and anteriorly, as seen on the axillary and Y-lateral views (B and C).

have three segments: head, both tuberosities, and shaft (Fig. 21A). In the "classic" four-part fracture, the head is dislocated out of the glenoid and devoid of any soft tissue attachment with tuberosities fragmented separately (Fig. 21B,C). In the "valgus-impacted" four-part fracture, the head is rotated to face upward with a remaining medial soft tissue hinge (Fig. 22).

If the head is split or has suffered an impaction fracture, it is considered to have articular loss (Fig. 23). Neer categorized these separately due to their poor prognosis and need for prosthetic replacement. Neer also categorized fracture-dislocations as two-, three-, or four-part fractures with either anterior or posterior dislocation of the articular segment.

In working with residents, we have found it useful to modify the Neer classification. In this system (Fig. 24) the direction of dislocation is not emphasized, isolated anatomic neck fractures are deleted since these are extremely rare, and four-part fractures have been separated into "classic" and "valgus impacted." By slightly simplifying the scheme, the essential aspects of the Neer classification may be better elucidated.

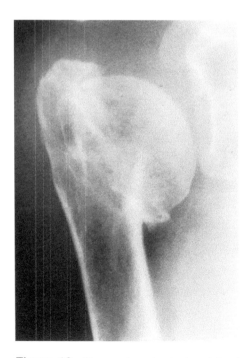

Figure 18   Two-part anatomical neck fracture. Uncommon variant shown on this AP view with early evidence of callous formation.

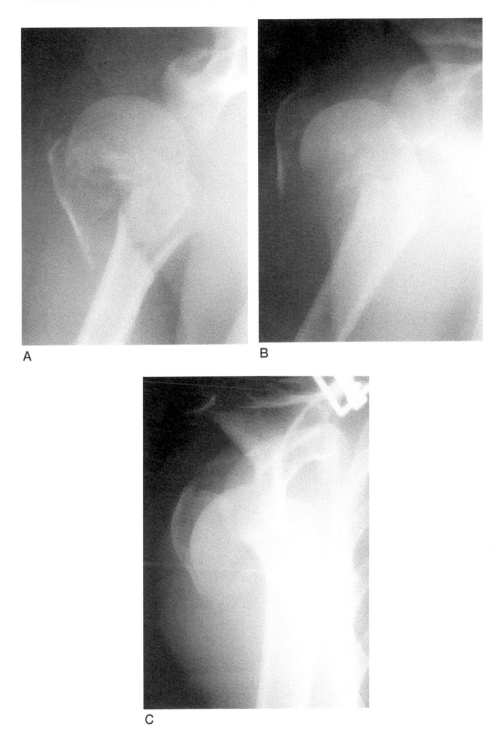

A

B

C

Figure 19 Three-part greater tuberosity fracture: includes displaced greater tuberosity and surgical neck fractures, which can be subtle in AP views (A) or more obvious (B). However, with a Y-lateral (C) view, the position of the parts can be better determined.

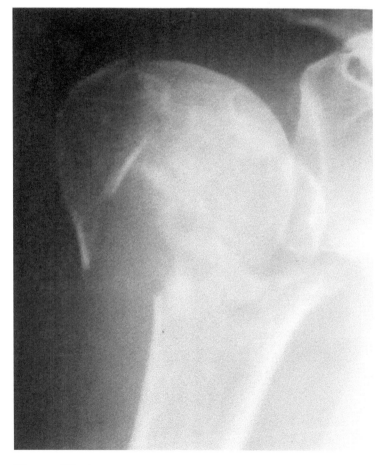

Figure 20 Three-part lesser tuberosity fracture. AP view shows medially displaced lesser tuberosity fragment with the head resting externally rotated.

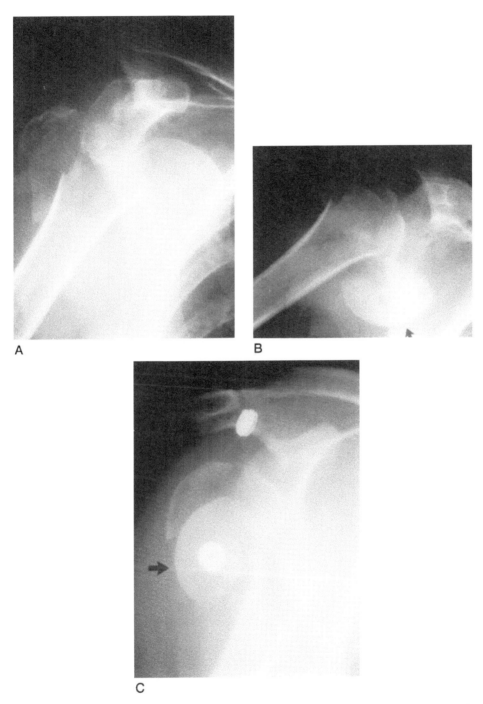

Figure 21 Four-part classic fracture: (A) AP view of this type of fracture in which the greater and lesser tuberosities remain attached to each other; (B) AP view of a classic four-part fracture in which the tuberosities are separated. In both, the head is dislocated into the axilla. (C) Four-part fracture Y-lateral view with the greater tuberosity fragment superior and posterior while the lesser tuberosity fragment and the humeral shaft are displaced anteriorly and medially.

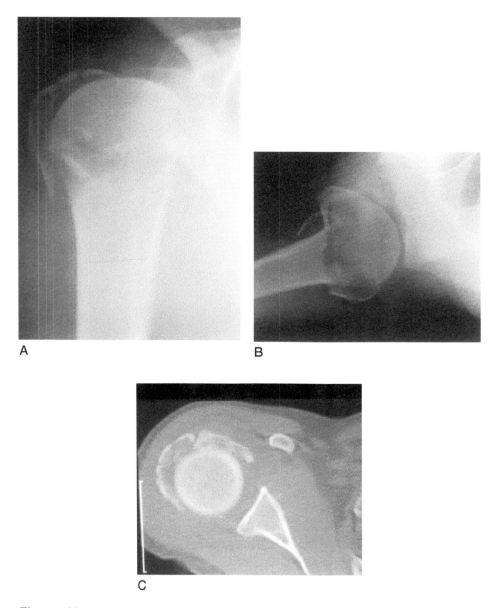

Figure 22 Four-part valgus-impacted fracture. (A) AP view with the head rotated superiorly in a nonarticulating position and both tuberosities displaced. In the axillary view (B) and the CT scan (C), the humeral head actually appears to articulate with the glenoid, again reinforcing the importance of obtaining views in different planes.

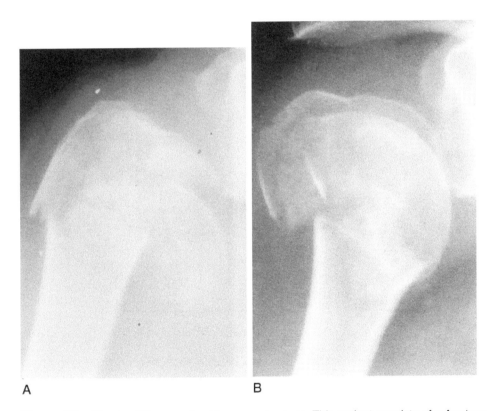

A   B

Figure 23 Head-splitting proximal humerus fracture. This variant consists of a fracture extending into a major portion of the articular surface as shown on both the AP-internal (A) and AP-external (B) views. View B shows the typical double density line.

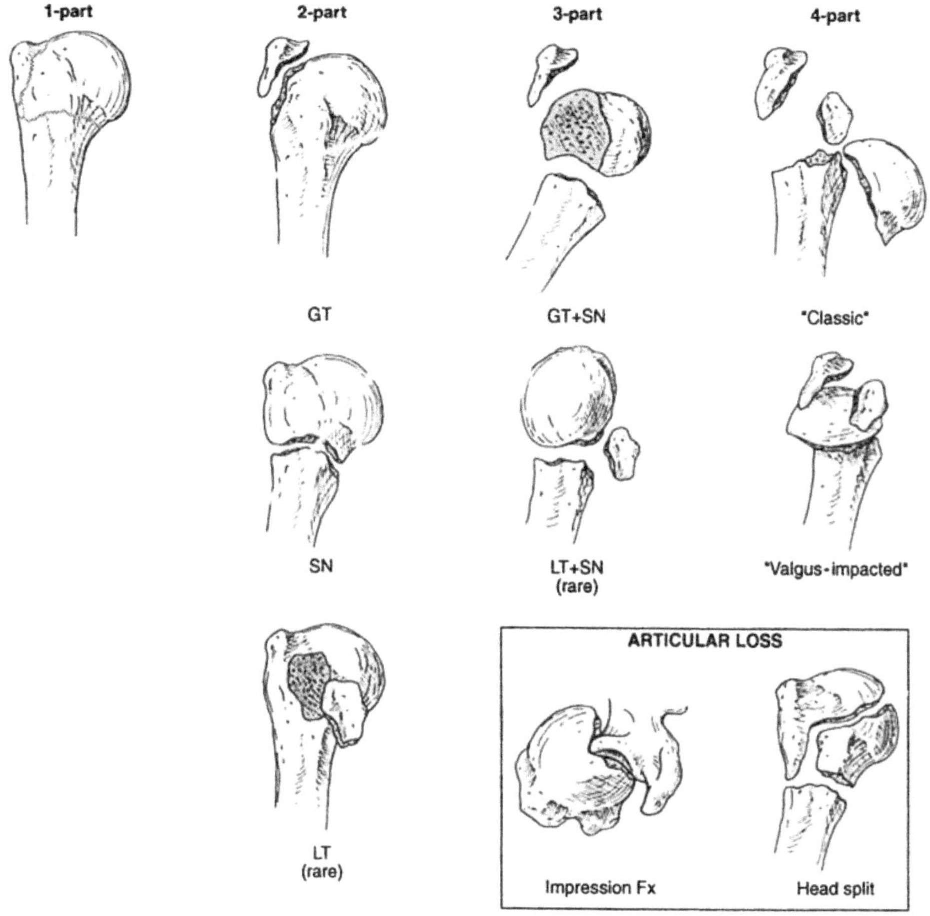

1-part	2-part	3-part	4-part
	GT	GT+SN	"Classic"
	SN	LT+SN (rare)	"Valgus-impacted"
LT (rare)			

ARTICULAR LOSS

Impression Fx   Head split

Figure 24 Simplified Neer classification system as described in text. The direction of location and anatomical neck fractures have been removed from the original Neer classification system. (From *Rockwood and Green's Fractures in Adults*, *5th ed.*, JD Heckman and RW Bucholz, eds. Philadelphia: Lippincott, Williams & Wilkins, 2001.)

VII CONCLUSION

Fracture displacement is a continuum, and good radiographs, experienced observers, and, in occasional cases, operative exploration may be needed for optimum classification. The classification schemes have evolved, and recently the validity of these descriptions has been questioned. The Neer classification system is still widely used by orthopedic surgeons for the diagnosis and treatment of proximal humeral fractures. It has reduced confusion in the literature by emphasizing the degree of displacement rather than the pattern of fracture lines. Furthermore, it provides the surgeon with a rationale for management and surgical planning based on the known fracture fragments and rotator cuff attachments (68).

REFERENCES

1. Benirschke SK, et al. Percutaneous pin fixation of surgical neck fractures of the humerus. Orthop Trans 1992; 16:231.

2. Bernstein J, et al. Evaluation of the Neer system of classification of proximal humeral fractures with computerized tomographic scans and plain radiographs. J Bone Joint Surg 1996; 78A:1371–1375.

3. Bixler BA, et al. Percutaneous pinning of proximal humerus fractures: a biomechanical study. Orthop Trans 1996; 20:865–866.

4. Blom S, Dahlback LO. Nerve injuries in dislocations of the shoulder joint and fractures of the neck of the humerus. A clinical and electromyographical study. Acta Chir Scand 1970; 136(6):461–466.

5. Bloom MH, Obata WG. Diagnosis of posterior dislocation of the shoulder with use of Velpeau axillary and angle-up roentgenographic views. J Bone Joint Surg (Am) 1967; 49(5):943–499.

6. Bohler J. Les fractures recentes de l'epaule. Acta Orthop Belg 1964; 30:235–242.

7. Boileau P, Walch G. The three-dimensional geometry of the proximal humerus. J Bone Joint Surg 1997; 79B(5):857–865.

8. Brooks CH, Revell WJ, Heatley FW. Vascularity of the humeral head after proximal humeral fractures. An anatomical cadaver study. J Bone Joint Surg Br 1993; 75(1):132–136.

9. Codman EA. The Shoulder: Rupture of the Supraspinatus Tendon and Other Lesions in or About the Subacromial Bursa. Boston: Thomas Todd, 1934.

10. De Anquin CE, De Anquin CA. Prosthetic replacement in the treatment of serious fractures of the proximal humerus. In: Bayley I, Kessel L, eds. Shoulder Surgery Berlin: Springer-Verlag, 1982:207–217.

11. Debevoise NT, Hyatt GW, Townsend GB. Humeral torsion in recurrent shoulder dislocations. A technic of determination by X-ray. Clin Orthop 1971; 76:87–93.

12. Dehne E. Fractures at the upper end of the humerus. Surg Clin North Am 1945; 25:28–47.

13. DePalma AF, Cautilli RA. Fractures of the upper end of the humerus. Clin Orthop Rel Res 1961; 20:73–93.

14. Esser J, et al. Detection of distant metastases of a phaeochromocytoma with 131I-metaiodobenzylguanidine. A case report. S Afr Med J 1984; 65(26):1057–1058.

15. Flatow EL, et al. Open reduction and internal fixation of two-part displaced fractures of the greater tuberosity of the proximal part of the humerus. J Bone Joint Surg (Am) 1991; 73(8):1213–1218.

16. Fourrier P, Martini M. Post-traumatic avascular necrosis of the humeral head. Int Orthop 1977; 1:187–190.

17. Galle P, et al. (Blood supply of the humeral head). Hefte Unfallheilkd 1975; (126):19–20.

18. Garceau GJ, Cogland S. Early physical therapy in the treatment of fractures of the surgical neck of the humerus. Indiana Med 1941; 34:293–295.

19. Gardener E. Innervation of the shoulder joint. Anat Rec 1948; 102:1–18.

20. Geneste R, et al. (The treatment of fracture-dislocation of the humeral head by blind pinning). Rev Chir Orthop Reparatrice Appar Mot 1980; 66(6):383–386.

21. Gerber C, Schneeberger AG, Vinh TS. The arterial vascularization of the humeral head. An anatomical study. J Bone Joint Surg (Am) 1990; 72(10):1486–1494.

22. Gold AM. Fractured neck of the humerus with separation and dislocation of the humeral head (fracture-dislocation of the shoulder, severe type). Bull Hosp Joint Dis 1971; 32(1):87–99.

23. Hagg O, Lundberg B. Aspects of prognostic factors in comminuted and dislocated proximal humeral fractures. In: Bateman JE, Welsh RP, eds. Surgery of the Shoulder. Philadelphia: B.C. Decker, 1984; 51–59.

24. Hall MC, Rosser M. The structure of the upper end of the humerus, with reference to osteoporotic changes in senescence leading to fractures. Can Med Assoc J 1963; 88:290–294.

25. Hardcastle PH, Fisher TR. Intrathoracic displacement of the humeral head with fracture of the surgical neck. Injury 1981; 12:313–315.

26. Hayes JM, Van Winkle GN. Axillary artery injury with minimally displaced fracture of the neck of the humerus. J Trauma 1983; 23(5):431–433.

27. Hill JA, Tkach L, Hendrix RW. A study of glenohumeral orientation in patients with anterior recurrent shoulder dislocations using computerized axial tomography. Orthop Rev 1989; 18(1):84–91.

28. Horak J, Nilsson B. Epidemiology of fractures of the upper end of the humerus. Clin Orthop Rel Res 1975; 112:250–253.

29. Hulke JW. Injuries of the upper extremity. In: Holmes T, ed. A System of Surgery, T. Holmes, New York: William Wood & Co, 1879: 764.

30. Jaberg H, Warner JJ, Jakob RP. Percutaneous stabilization of unstable fractures of the humerus. J Bone Joint Surg (Am) 1992; 74(4):508–515.

31. Jakob RP, et al. Four-part valgus impacted fractures of the proximal humerus. J Bone Joint Surg (Br) 1991; 73(2):295–298.

32. Kelly JP. Fractures complicating electroconvulsive therapy and chronic epilepsy. J Bone Joint Surg 1954; 36B:70–79.

33. Knight RA, Mayne JA. Comminuted fractures and fracture-dislocations involving the articular surface of the humeral head. J Bone Joint Surg 1957; 39A:1343–1355.

34. Kocher MS, Dupre MM, Feagin JA Jr. Shoulder injuries from alpine skiing and snowboarding. Aetiology, treatment and prevention. Sports Med 1998; 25(3):201–211.

35. Kocher MS, Feagin JA Jr. Shoulder injuries during alpine skiing. Am J Sports Med 1996; 24(5):665–669.

36. Kocher T. Beiträge zur Kenntnis einiger Praktisch Wichtiger Frakturformen. Basel: Carl Sallmann, 1896.

37. Kofoed H. Revascularization of the humeral head. A report of two cases of fracture-dislocation of the shoulder. Clin Orthop 1983; (179):175–178.

38. Krahl V. The torsion of the humerus: its localization, cause, and duration in man. Am J Anat 1947; 80:275–319.

39. Kristiansen B, et al. The Neer classification of fractures of the proximal humerus. An assessment of interobserver variation. Skel Radiol 1988; 17(6):420–422.

40. Kronberg M, Brostrom LA, Soderlund V. Retroversion of the humeral head in the normal shoulder and its relationship to the normal range of motion. Clin Orthop 1990; (253):113–117.

41. Laing PG. The arterial supply of the adult humerus. J Bone Joint Surg 1956; 38A:1105–1116.

42. Lind T, Kroner K, Jensen J. The epidemiology of fractures of the proximal humerus. Arch Orthop Trauma Surg 1989; 108(5):285–287.

43. Meeder PJ, Wiese K, Wentzensen A. Results of an operative therapy of dislocated fractures of the humeral head in adults. Aktuel Traumatol 1980; 10:201.

44. Meyerding HW. Fracture-dislocation of the shoulder. Minn Med 1937; 20:717–726.

45. Moseley HF, Goldie I. The arterial pattern of the rotator cuff and the shoulder. J Bone Joint Surg 1963; 45B:780–789.

46. Muller ME, et al. The Comprehensive Classification of Fractures of Long Bones. Berlin: Springer-Verlag, 1990.

47. Neer CS. Articular replacement for the humeral head. J Bone Joint Surg 1955; 37A:215–228.

48. Neer CS, Borwn TH, McLaughlin HL. Fracture of the neck of the humerus with dislocation of the head fragment. Am J Surg 1953; 85:252–258.

49. Neer CSD. Displaced proximal humeral fractures. I. Classification and evaluation. J Bone Joint Surg (Am) 1970; 52(6):1077–1089.

50. Neer CSD. Displaced proximal humeral fractures. II. Treatment of three-part and four-part displacement. J Bone Joint Surg (Am) 1970; 52(6):1090–1103.

51. Pieper HG. Shoulder dislocation in skiing: choice of surgical method depending on the degree of humeral retrotorsion. Int J Sports Med 1985; 6(3):155–160.

52. Randelli M, Gambrioli PL. Glenohumeral osteometry by computed tomography in normal and unstable shoulders. Clin Orthop 1986; (208):151–156.

53. Rechtman AM. Open reduction of fracture dislocation of the humerus. J Am Med Assoc 1930; 94:1656–1657.

54. Resch H, Beck E, Bayley I. Reconstruction of the valgus-impacted humeral head fracture. J Shoulder Elbow Surg 1995; 4(2):73–80.

55. Rose SH, et al. Epidemiologic features of humeral fractures. Clin Orthop 1982; 64(168):24–30.

56. Rothman RH, Parke WW. The vascular anatomy of the rotator cuff. Clin Orthop 1965; 41:176–186.

57. Saitoh S, Nakatsuchi Y. Osteoporosis of the proximal humerus: comparison of bone mineral density and mechanical strength with the proximal femur. J Shoulder Elbow Surg 1993; 2:78–84.

58. Saitoh S, et al. Distribution of bone mineral density and bone strength of the proximal humerus. J Shoulder Elbow Surg 1994; 3:234–242.

59. Salem MI. Bilateral anterior fracture-dislocation of the shoulder joints due to severe electric shock. Injury 1983; 14:361–363.

60. Sidor ML, et al. The Neer classification system for proximal humeral fractures. An assessment of interobserver reliability and intraobserver reproducibility. J Bone Joint Surg Am 1993; 75(12):1745–1750.

61. Siebenrock KA, Gerber C. The reproducibility of classification of fractures of the proximal end of the humerus. J Bone Joint Surg Am 1993; 75(12):1751–1755.

62. Sjoden GO, et al. Poor reproducibility of classification of proximal humeral fractures. Additional CT of minor value. Acta Orthop Scand 1997; 68(3):239–242.

63. Stableforth PG. Four-part fractures of the neck of the humerus. J Bone Joint Surg (Br) 1984; 66(1):104–108.

64. Sturzenegger M, Fornaro E, Jakob RP. Results of surgical treatment of multifragmented fractures of the humeral head. Arch Orthop Trauma Surg 1982; 100(4):249–259.

65. Svend-Hansen H. Displaced proximal humeral fractures. A review of 49 patients. Acta Orthop Scand 1974; 45(3):359–364.

66. Tillet E, et al. Anatomic determination of humeral head retroversion: the relationship of the central axis of the humeral head to the bicipital groove. J Shoulder Elbow Surg, 1993; 2:255–256.

67. Watson-Jones R. Fracture of the neck of the humerus. In: Fractures and Other Bone and Joint Injuries. Baltimore: Williams and Wilkens, 1940; 289–297.

68. Williams GR Jr, Wong KL. Two-part and three-part fractures: open reduction and internal fixation versus closed reduction and percutaneous pinning. Orthop Clin North Am 2000; 31(1):1–21.

69. Zuckerman JD, et al. Axillary artery injury as a complication of proximal humeral fractures. Two case reports and a review of the literature. Clin Orthop 1984; 189:234–237.

70. Bigliani, Flatow. The Shoulder: Operative Techniques. Philadelphia: Williams and Wilkins, 1998.
71. Ianotti, Williams. Disorders of the Shoulder. Philidelphia: Lippincott, Williams and Wilkins, 1999.

2

Percutaneous Treatment of Proximal Humeral Fractures

HERBERT RESCH and CLEMENS HÜBNER

General Hospital Salzburg, Salzburg, Austria

I INTRODUCTION

Nonoperative treatment of displaced humeral head fractures does not lead to satisfying results (1–4). Reduction of the fragments is therefore essential, although there is a danger that reduction by open surgery may increase the risk of avascular necrosis (AVN) in four-part fractures and four-part fracture dislocations. The risk of AVN is increased further, however, by exposure of the fracture as required for plating osteosynthesis in comparison to the exposure required for minimal osteosynthesis (5–7). Open minimal osteosynthesis is therefore the treatment of choice, at least in younger people, due to the fact that the survival time of a prosthetic implant is limited (5,6). In order to avoid the additional risk of AVN involved in open surgery, percutaneous treatment is an even more desirable procedure.

Minimally invasive surgery for humeral head fractures began in 1962, when Böhler first described percutaneously inserted pins for the fixation of unstable subcapital fractures (8). This treatment was later also recommended by other authors, but only for minimally displaced three-part fractures (5,6,9). Svend-Hansen and Stableforth reported unsatisfactory results with this method, but neither provided the details of their technique (3,4). At the very least it can be said that percutaneous reduction and fixation does not increase the risk of AVN and would therefore be a desirable method of treatment. The questions that arise with this kind of treatment are (1) whether anatomical reduction can be achieved by this method and (2) how the achieved result can be maintained percutaneously. The latter question on fixation is especially important in patients with osteoporotic bone.

33

II PREOPERATIVE ASSESSMENT AND PLANNING

A thorough understanding of the anatomical relationships among the various fragments is extremely important not only for the blood supply of the humeral head but also to benefit from the so-called ligamentotaxis effect (5). Therefore it is important to study the "personality" of the fracture in detail before operating. An intact periosteum can be used to the surgeon's advantage, and careful inspection of the fracture pattern will help determine the integrity of the periosteum. For example, if a fracture occurs but there is no distance between the two fragments, it can be assumed that the periosteum is still intact. On the other hand, the greater the distance between the fragments, the greater the likelihood that the periosteum is destroyed or stripped off from the bone. In cases where the head fragment is displaced medially or laterally in relation to the shaft, the periosteum can be injured in two areas. When the head fragment is displaced medially, the periosteum will be stripped off from the shaft fragment but up to a certain amount of displacement will not be destroyed. This is also true with respect to the vessels within the periosteum. When the head is displaced laterally, however, the periosteum then runs over the sharp edge of the shaft fragment and will be destroyed much sooner than with medial displacement (Fig. 1). Based on anatomical and biomechanical studies, rupture of the periostum begins on average after 9 mm with medial displacement and after 6 mm with lateral displacement (10). At that time it is still unknown up to which amount of displacement blood flow in the tensioned periosteum still occurs and when it is stopped. Currently, studies are still ongoing to determine these critical issues. Displacement of the humeral head usually does not occur in the horizontal direction only but is combined with additional displacement of the head segment in the posterior direction.

A carefully performed preoperative examination of the fractured head is mandatory. Visualization on at least two x-ray views (antero-posterior and axillary

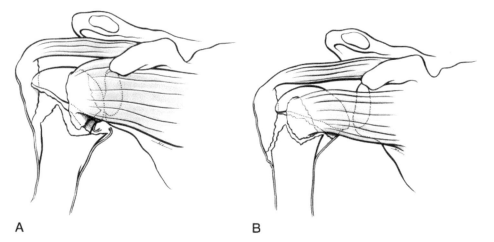

A   B

Figure 1 Four-part fracture with horizontal displacement of articular segment. (A) Marked lateral displacement of articular segment, periosteum on medial side destroyed, on lateral side stripped off but not destroyed. (B) Marked medial displacement of articular segment, periosteum on medial side stripped off but not destroyed, on lateral side intact.

view) is crucial for correct fracture assessment. It is recommended to perform an additional transscapular view (Neer Trauma series) (2). The personality of the fracture is best demonstrated with three-dimensional (3D) computed tomography (CT) reconstruction. This is especially useful for percutaneous treatment.

III INDICATIONS/CONTRAINDICATIONS

Percutaneous pinning is a preferable method of treatment for extra-articular humeral head fractures, including the greater tuberosity and subcapital region. In addition, certain indications for intra-articular fractures may be considered.

Good indications include:

1. Surgical neck fractures with avulsion of the greater tuberosity [three-part fractures (Neer); B1and B21- (AO classification) (11,12)]
2. Impacted humeral head fractures without severe lateral displacement [valgus impacted four-part fractures; C1 and C2 (AO)]

Lesser indications include:

1. Humeral head fractures with severe lateral displacement of the articular segment ["true" four-part fractures (Neer), some types of C2 (AO)]
2. Severely displaced fracture dislocations [VI (Neer); C3 (AO)]

It is always possible to attempt percutaneous methods even in situations with poorer indications. However, one should always be prepared to convert to an open approach if adequate reduction and fixation cannot be achieved.

IV TECHNIQUE

A Instruments

Reduction is performed with a percutaneously inserted elevator and a pointed hook retractor. Maintenance of the reduction is performed with 2.2 mm Kirschner wires (K-wires). Within the last 3 years, a K-wire locking screw with a guide system for the introduction of the K-wires was developed to avoid K-wire migration (Humerus-block, F/O group). The idea of this locking screw is not only to avoid migration of the K-wires, but also to obtain stable fixation of the K-wires in the cortex of the shaft and in the locking screw as well. This avoids displacement of the head in any direction but allows the head segment to glide in the direction of the K-wires in order to settle on the shaft fragment, which leads to rapid healing (so-called "guided sliding" of the head).

Screw fixation of the tuberosities is performed with a cannulated screw fixation system (Leibinger, Freiburg, Germany).

B Patient Positioning

The operation is usually performed under regional anesthesia. The patient is placed in the supine position with the upper body inclined at an angle of about 30° (Fig. 2). The patient's head is supported on a headrest. The arm is draped to permit mobility. The image intensifier is located cranially. The C-arm is set to create a right angle between the central beam and the humeral head and shaft, respectively. During the

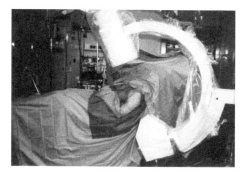

Figure 2 Positioning of patient. Patient in supine position with upper body in about 30° of upright position. Patient's arm draped free, intensifier in cranial position, upper arm right-angled to central beam.

operation the surgeons wear special radioresistent gloves (Fluoro-shield Radiation Reduction Gloves, Smith & Nephew Inc., Andover, MA).

C Landmarks

Orientation of the humeral head in the cranio-caudal direction is provided by the image intensifier, while for antero-posterior (AP) orientation the humeral head is divided into thirds with a marker pen. For this purpose the surgeon places his thumb and index finger on the anterior and posterior sides of the humeral head and squeezes hard. The distance between the two fingers corresponds to the AP extension of the humeral head, which is then divided into thirds. With the humeral head in a neutral position, the transition between the anterior and middle third corresponds roughly to the intertubercular groove.

D Fracture of the Greater Tuberosity

Fractures of the greater tuberosity can be differentiated by the pathomechanics of the injury into three types:

1. Isolated fractures
2. Fractures associated with shoulder dislocation
3. Fractures in conjunction with complex humeral head fracture

Isolated fractures are caused by the pull of the tendons of the rotator cuff muscles and are usually seen in younger patients when tendons are stronger than the bone. The fragment is usually displaced in superior-posterior direction into the subacromial space since the periosteum between the fragment and shaft is destroyed (Fig. 3).

Following an anterior shoulder dislocation, the greater tuberosity is avulsed by the pull of the tendons of the supraspinatus, specifically the infraspinatus muscle. The periosteum on the posterior side remains intact, whereas it ruptures on the lateral side. After reduction of the dislocated head, the tuberosity remains posteriorly displaced, but is not displaced cranially. The reduction may appear near-anatomical

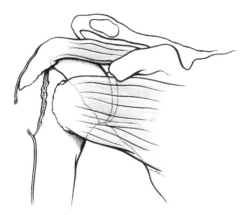

Figure 3   Isolated avulsion fracture of the greater tuberosity. Periosteum between shaft and fragment is destroyed and the tuberosity is displaced into the subacromial space by the pull of the supra- and infraspinatus muscles.

in the AP view, but this can be misleading since posterior displacement rarely is identified with this projection.

Greater tuberosity fractures associated with complex fractures can be categorized as follows:

1. Complex fractures in which the shaft fragment is still in axial alignment with the humeral head fragment. The fracture of the tuberosity is caused indirectly by the depression of the articular head fragment. In these cases the tuberosity is displaced just laterally and perhaps slightly posteriorly but never superiorly as the periosteum between tuberosity and shaft remains intact (see Fig.7).
2. Complex fractures in which the shaft fragment is not in axial alignment with the head fragment. Depending on the amount of medial displacement of the shaft fragment, the periosteum between tuberosity and shaft is destroyed. In this case the tuberosity is displaced in superior and posterior direction caused by the pull of the adherent muscles (see Fig. 6).

The technique of reduction and fixation of isolated fractures of the greater tuberosity (with superior displacement) is shown in Figure 4. The patient's arm is held in a neutral position by the assistant. A small incision is made at the limit of the anterior and middle third of the humeral head about 1 cm below the superior border of the tuberosity and a small but sturdy hook retractor is introduced in the direction of the fibers through the deltoid muscle and into the subacromial space. The subacromial space is enlarged by applying slight traction to the arm. The tuberosity is engaged at the insertion of the supraspinatus tendon and moved anteriorly and caudally until the correct position appears to have been reached, i.e., the profile of the head is normal.

Temporary fixation of the tuberosity in this position is performed either with a 2 mm K-wire or with the drill-guidewire combination (Cannulated Screw Fixation System, Oswald Leibinger, Freiburg, Germany), which is 2.2 mm thick. The correct

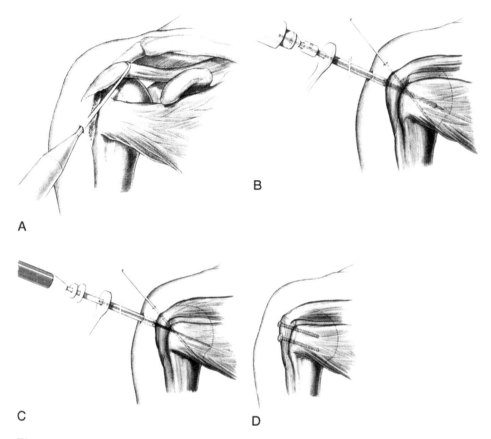

Figure 4 Technique of percutaneous reconstruction of greater tuberosity. (A) The pointed hook retractor is inserted via a stab incision at the transition zone between anterior and medial third and about 1 cm below the original height of the tuberosity. The fragment is grasped at the insertion of the supraspinatus tendon and pulled in a downward and slightly anterior direction. (B) The tuberosity is secured temporarily with either a K-wire or directly with the drill-guidewire combination. Then the arm is rotated internally and externally to check the position of the tuberosity. (C) The drill is removed and the guide wire remains in place. Forty mm long cannulated self-tapping screws are introduced over the guidewire. (D) The tuberosity is fixed with two screws.

position of the tuberosity is checked by maximal internal and external rotation of the arm. With the arm in slight internal rotation (10–15°), a cannula with the blunt trocar is inserted through the deltoid muscle toward the greater tuberosity via an incision placed on the transition zone of the middle and posterior third of the AP diameter of the head. The trocar is advanced until it is just in contact with the profile of the tuberosity, i.e., there is no bone-metal overlap under image intensifier control. The correct position on the bony profile is confirmed by sliding the trocar from a slight anterior to posterior direction. This reveals the correct insertion point for the drill-guidewire combination and the screw in the AP direction without having to relocate the image intensifier from the AP alignment.

The cannula is pressed against the tuberosity, the blunt trocar removed, and the drill-guidewire combination is drilled in place to the maximum depth permitted by the depth gauge on the drill (40 mm). The guidewire is released and a driver used to tap it in to improve the anchorage in the bone. The drill is extracted manually, leaving the guidewire behind. A 40 mm cannulated titanium self-tapping screw is then screwed in place. The screw is usually used without a washer to avoid metal impingement on the acromion and possible axillary nerve entrapment. A washer is used only in cases with a comminuted tuberosity. One to three screws are applied depending on the size of the fragment.

E   Anatomical Neck Fractures

Anatomical neck fractures (Fig. 5) are rare compared to surgical neck fractures as well as three- and four-part fractures. In anatomical neck fractures the head fragment is usually shifted medially and slightly posteriorly. The elevator is inserted percutaneously via a stab incision, and it is directed anterior to the humeral head and kept in contact with the bone of the humeral head leading to the anatomical neck. The anatomical neck is then pushed superiorly while traction is applied to the slightly abducted arm, which is in neutral rotational position. In case of additional posterior displacement, the shaft fragment has to be pushed backwards at the same time while the head is pushed superiorly. The reduced head tensions the rotator cuff, which causes the greater tuberosity to approximate to the normal anatomical site.

F   Surgical Neck Fractures with Avulsion of the Greater Tuberosity (Three-Part Fracture)

In severely displaced fractures, the head is rotated internally by the pull of the subscapularis muscle, which is not counteracted by the infraspinatus muscle because of the fracture of the greater tuberosity (Fig. 6). Additionally, the shaft is displaced anteriorly and medially. These fractures are usually very unstable because all soft tissue links between the shaft and head have been disrupted. The greater tuberosity displaces into the subacromial space and has also lost its periosteal connections to the shaft. Therefore, both fragments have to be reduced with a separate maneuver.

First the subcapital fracture is reduced with the arm in adduction and internal rotation with simultaneous traction applied to the arm and the surgeon using his thumb to apply counterpressure towards postero-lateral in the area of the fracture. The fracture is then secured by means of three 2.2 mm K-wires drilled from inferiorly to superiorly through the fragment of the humeral shaft. Then the arm is returned carefully to the neutral position and the greater tuberosity reduced by means of the pointed hook retractor inserted into the subacromial space. The greater tuberosity is engaged at the insertion of the supraspinatus tendon and moved antero-inferiorly until the correct position appears to have been reached. After temporary fixation with a K-wire, the correct position of the tuberosity is checked by maximum external and internal rotation of the arm. Finally, the tuberosity is fixed by means of two cannulated titanium screws. In cases of pronounced rotational displacement, a hook is inserted and the lesser tuberosity grasped at the insertion area of the subscapularis tendon to achieve derotation of the head. When the profile of the humeral head appears normal, the K-wires are inserted through the shaft.

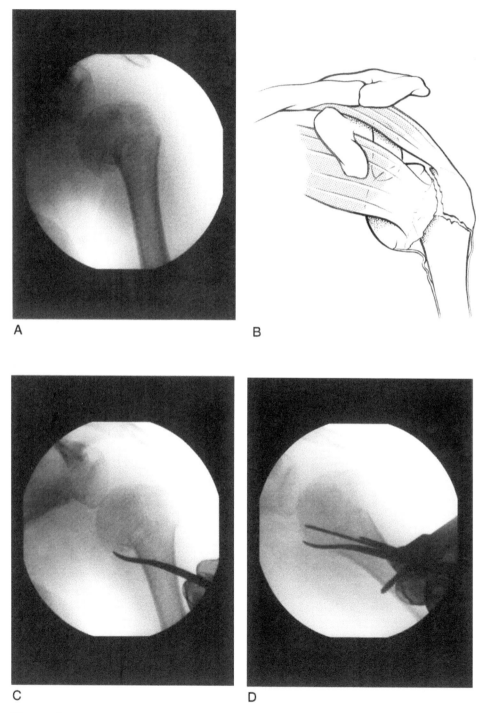

A

B

C

D

Figure 5 Anatomical neck fracture. (A) Head fragment is shifted medially and inferiorly. The greater tuberosity is fractured but almost undisplaced. (B) Drawing depicting part A.

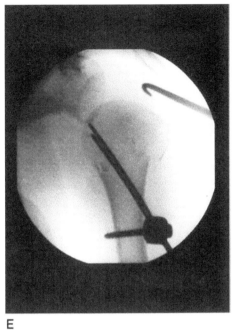
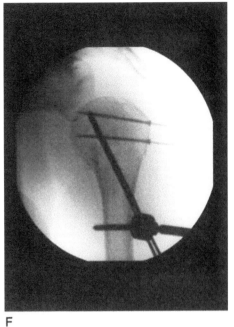

E

F

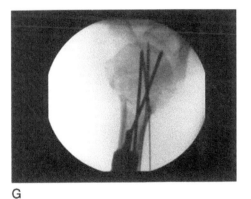

G

Caused by the medial and inferior shift of the head, it can be assumed that the periosteum on the medial side is stripped off but not destroyed (see also Fig. 1).The periosteum on the lateral side is undestroyed. (C) Elevator inserted through stab incision and led along the bone to medial and inferior part of articular segment. (D) Articular segment reduced by superior movement using the elevator. K-wires, which have been introduced before through the cortex of the shaft, are drilled into the head at the right moment of reduction. (E) Greater tuberosity is slightly displaced posteriorly and is reduced using the hook retractor, elevator, and/or the drill-guidewire combination. (F) Articular segment fixed by two K-wires, which are locked in the Humerusblock. Greater tuberosity is fixed by two cannulated screws. (G) Axial view; satisfactory reduction, lesser tuberosity not fractured.

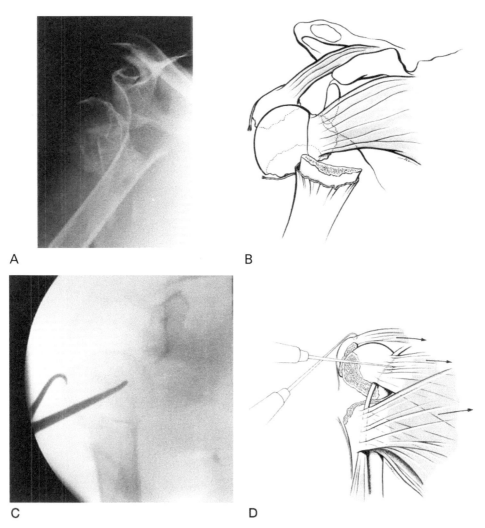

A   B

C   D

Figure 6   Three-part fracture of a 78-year-old woman with fracture of the surgical neck and the greater tuberosity but unfractured lesser tuberosity. (A) Complete separation of head and shaft fragment which is displaced far medially. Greater tuberosity is displaced superiorly. Head is rotated internally. Lesser tuberosity not fractured. (B) Drawing depicting part A. All periostal connections between head and shaft and greater tuberosity and shaft are interrupted. Shaft is displaced medially by the pull of the pectoral major muscle. Greater tuberosity is displaced superiorly and posteriorly by the supra- and infraspinatus. Subscapularis is not counteracted by the infraspinatus, resulting in internal rotation of the head. Highly unstable fracture. (C) The head fragment is derotated by means of a pointed hook retractor until the profile of the head looks normal. With a second hook retractor, the greater tuberosity is reduced in downward and slight anterior direction. With the head held in this position, the shaft is brought in alignment with the head. (D) Drawing depicting part C. First, the head is derotated by means of a hook retractor, which is engaged at the insertion of the subscapularis; second, the greater tuberosity is reduced with a second hook retractor engaged at the insertion of the supraspinatus. (E) The head is fixed with two K-wires, which are locked in the so-called Humerusblock. The tuberosity is fixed with cannulated self-tapping screws.

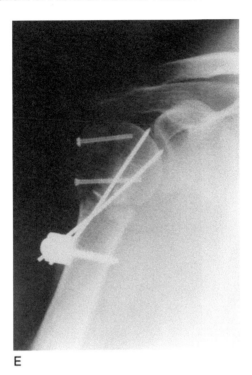

E

G Surgical Neck Fractures with Avulsion of the Lesser Tuberosity (Three-Part Fracture)

In these fractures the shaft fragment is usually displaced far medially by the pull of the pectoral major muscle (Fig. 7). The fractured lesser tuberosity is displaced medially by the pull of the subscapularis muscle. All the periosteal connections between head and shaft and head and lesser tuberosity are interrupted. The greater tuberosity is not fractured, and due to the pull of the supra- and infraspinatus muscles the head is rotated into the varus position.

Reduction is performed in a similar fashion as detailed above. First, a stab incision is made and an elevator is used to correct the varus deformity by pushing the head medially. At the same time, the subcapital fracture is reduced by bringing the shaft in alignment with the head. The shaft fragment is kept in slight abduction and neutral rotation. Previously placed K-wires are then directed into the head from the shaft. (The K-wires should be placed into the shaft and left there so that after the reduction is achieved, the surgeon need only advance the wires into the head.) Finally, the lesser tuberosity, which is usually displaced medially, has to be reduced. For this purpose the patient's arm is held in 70° of abduction, and the image intensifier is set for an axial view. A small incision is made and the hook retractor advanced towards the lesser tuberosity, which is engaged at the insertion area of

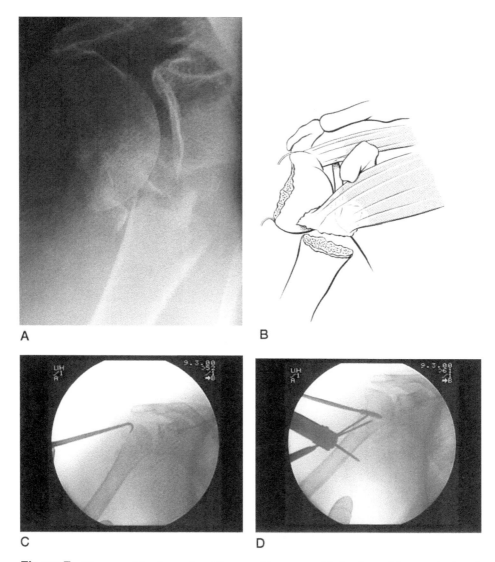

A   B

C   D

Figure 7   Three-part fracture of an 82-year-old woman with fracture of the surgical neck and the lesser tuberosity but unfractured greater tuberosity. (A) Complete separation of head and shaft fragment; the latter is displaced far medially. Lesser tuberosity is fractured and displaced medially. The greater tuberosity is unfractured. The head is rotated in a clockwise direction into varus position. (B) Drawing depicting part A. No periostal links between head and shaft and head and lesser tuberosity as well. The shaft is displaced far medially by the pectoral major muscle. The lesser tuberosity is pulled medially by the subscapularis muscle. Due to the unfractured greater tuberosity, the supra- and infraspinatus muscles are still active and not counteracted by either periostal links between head and shaft on the inferior side or the subscapularis, resulting in varus deformity of head. (C) Head is derotated by means of a hook retractor and the shaft fragment is brought into alignment with the head. (D) "Prepared" K-wires are "waiting" for insertion into the head at the right moment when reduction is achieved. Additional reduction with the elevator. (E) K-wires are blocked in the Humerusblock. (F) Reduction of lesser tuberosity. The shaft is abducted up to 70°. The lesser tuberosity, which is displaced far medially, is reduced with an

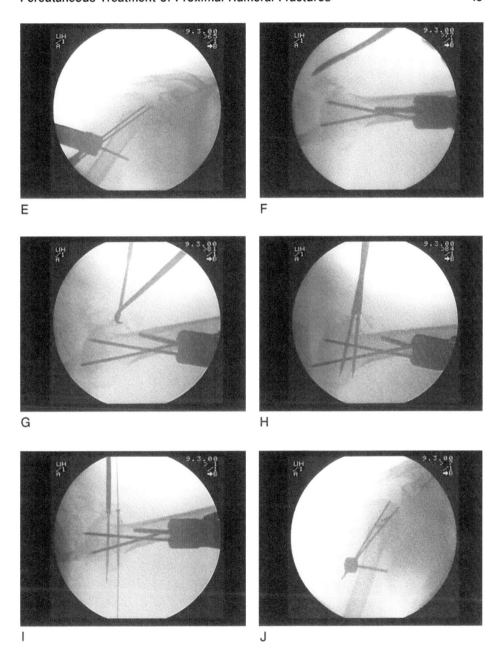

E

F

G

H

I

J

elevator or a hook retractor. (G) The lesser tuberosity is pulled laterally with a hook retractor, which is engaged at the insertion of the lesser tuberosity until the step formation of the articular surface has disappeared. The drill is inserted for temporary fixation. (H) The fragment is secured temporarily with two drills or K-wires. (I) Lesser tuberosity is fixed with two cannulated screws which are inserted over the guide wire. (J) Head is fixed with two K-wires and lesser tuberosity with two screws. Due to the very porotic bone quality, the tips of the K-wires are drilled through the subchondral bone to find a better grip. (K) Fracture 4 months after accident; K-wires were removed after 6 weeks and withdrawn after 3 weeks under local anesthesia.

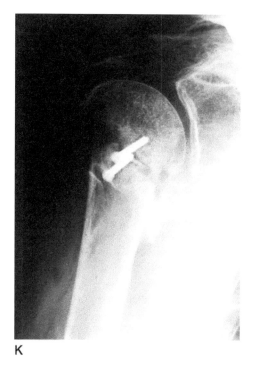

K

Figure 7 Continued.

subscapularis tendon and pulled laterally until the articular incongruity seen medially disappears. Temporary fixation is provided with the drill guide wire combination or a K-wire, and a 40 mm screw is placed anteroposteriorly. Finally the K-wires initially drilled into the head segment are cut off and left just beneath the skin.

H Valgus-Impacted Fractures (Valgus-Impacted Four-Part Fractures)

In these fractures (Fig. 8) the head segment is impacted into the metaphysis with or without additional lateral or medial displacement. The greater tuberosity is displaced laterally but remains in the correct longitudinal position. The lesser tuberosity is displaced anteriorly and remains also in the correct longitudinal position but is usually slightly displaced medially by the pull of the subscapularis. Because the tuberosities are not displaced in the longitudinal direction, the periosteum remains mostly intact (the periosteum may be slightly stripped off the shaft). If the head is not displaced medially or laterally, the periosteum on the medial side of the anatomical neck is not destroyed. This is important not only because of the blood supply to the head segment but because it can also be used as a mechanical "hinge" (so-called hinge periosteum) when the head is raised.

The principles of reduction are the same as with the open technique. Reconstruction involves raising the head segment, as that is the only way to restore

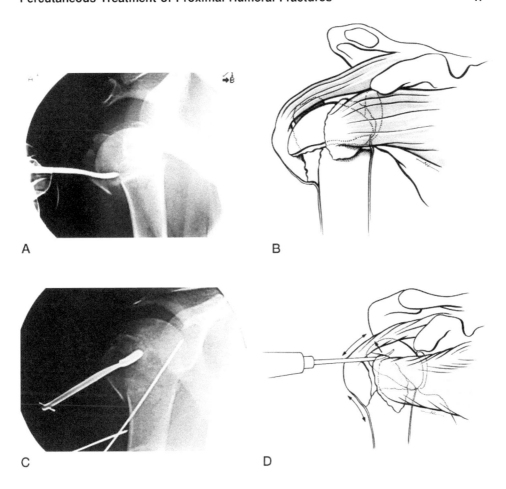

A   B

C   D

Figure 8 Valgus-impacted four-part fracture (A) The humeral head is deeply depressed into the metaphysis without marked horizontal displacement. Greater tuberosity fractured with only lateral displacement, which is caused by the articular segment but no superior displacement. Lesser tuberosity is fractured but only minimally displaced. (B) Drawing depicting part A. Due to the lack of horizontal displacement, it can be assumed that the periosteum on the medial side is not destroyed (intact "hinge" periosteum). As the greater tuberosity is not displaced superiorly, it can be assumed that the periosteum between greater tuberosity and the shaft is not destroyed, perhaps slightly stripped off from the shaft. The same is true with the lesser tuberosity. As it is not displaced medially by the subscapularis, it can be assumed that the periosteum between shaft and lesser tuberosity is still intact. (C) Head is raised by means of an elevator and K-wires are inserted at the right time of reduction. Fixation is performed as described above. (D) Drawing depicting part C. The elevator is introduced via the intertubercular fracture gap, which is ∼ 5–10 mm lateral to the bicipital groove. The articular head fragment is raised by the elevator using the intact medial periosteum as a hinge ("hinge-periosteum").The reduced head causes tensioning of the rotator cuff and tensioning of the lateral periosteum, which on its side causes reduction of the greater tuberosity.

the anatomy of the tuberosities. The patient's arm is held in adduction and neutral rotation by the surgeon's assistant. An incision is made on the junction between the anterior and middle thirds of the head, and, working under image intensifier control, an elevator is advanced towards the impacted articular segment. The fracture gap between the two tuberosities, which almost always occupies the same location (about 5–10 mm lateral to the bicipital groove), is located by gently sliding the tip of the elevator over the bone in the AP direction. Through this gap the elevator is inserted into the fracture below the humeral head. The segment is then raised to the anatomical position, as indicated by the greater tuberosity. The reduced head segment is secured with two or three 2.2 mm K-wires drilled from inferiorly through the fragment of the shaft into the articular segment. The greater tuberosity, which is tilted laterally due to the impaction, normally reduces anatomically when the articular segment is raised. It is held inferiorly by the residual periosteum and superiorly by the rotator cuff. The cannula of the screw fixation system with the blunt trocar is advanced towards the upper part of the greater tuberosity, and a screw is inserted through the tuberosity into the upper part of the articular segment. Another screw is passed through the inferior part of the greater tuberosity into the fragment of the shaft so that the greater tuberosity has fixation to both the shaft and the articular segment. Reduction and fixation of the lesser tuberosity is performed as described above.

I Severely Displaced Humeral Head Fractures ("True" Four-Part Fractures and Four-Part Fracture-Dislocation)

The head fragment is displaced far away from the shaft fragment, and very little or no soft tissue links exist anymore (destroyed hinge periosteum). The extreme variant of this fracture type is the four-part fracture-dislocation. Percutaneous as well as open reduction is very difficult to obtain, and because the risk of AVN is high, prosthetic replacement would be the treatment of choice in these cases. In younger patients an attempt, closed or open, should be made to reduce the fracture in order to obtain reasonable anatomy of the humeral head. If AVN does develop, a good functional outcome can be expected with prosthetic replacement.

In some elderly patients in which the condition of the patient does not allow the implantation of a prosthesis, an attempt of percutaneous treatment, performed under regional anesthesia, can be made (Fig. 9).

1 Exposure to Radiation

Average exposure time during operation was slightly more than 7 minutes for the first five patients. However, the exposure time decreased to 3 minutes in subsequent patients.

2 Postoperative Management

The arm is immobilized against the body with light bandages for 3 weeks. Depending on the degree of stability achieved, passive exercise in the plane of the scapula without rotation is started on the first postoperative day. In the fourth week of therapy, rotation and active movement exercises are started. After 4–6 weeks, the K-wires are removed with local anesthesia. Radiographs with AP and transscapular views are performed 1, 3, 6, and 12 weeks postoperative and after 1 year.

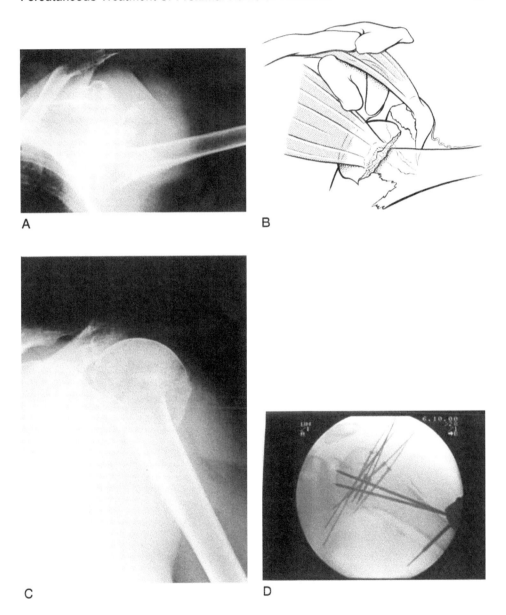

A   B

C   D

Figure 9 Four-part fracture dislocation in an 86-year-old woman. (A) Articular segment almost separated from shaft fragment, greater tuberosity still in contact with shaft, lesser tuberosity displaced medially. (B) Drawing depicting part B. Periosteal connections only on the postero-medial part of the articular segment and between shaft and greater tuberosity. (C) After closed reduction the fracture is changed into a valgus-type four-part fracture. (D) The head was raised by means of an elevator. The greater and lesser tuberosities were reduced using the hook retractor and the elevator according to the technique shown in Figures 6 and 7. Due to the porotic bone quality, the tips of the K-wires are drilled through the subchondral bone in order to achieve a better grip. The K-wires are withdrawn after 3 weeks under local anesthesia when moving exercises are started. (E) X-ray at the end of surgery. (F) X-ray after removal of K-wires.

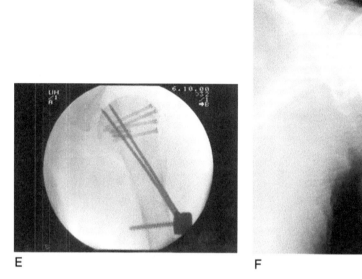

E   F

Figure 9   Continued.

V   RESULTS

Between 1990 and 1994, 27 patients with three-part and four-part fractures (9 and 18 patients, respectively) were treated using the percutaneous technique for reduction and screw fixation (13). Of the 18 patients with four-part fractures, 13 were of the valgus type without any significant lateral displacement of the articular segment, while 5 showed significant displacement. Near-anatomical restoration of the humeral head was achieved with almost all fractures. The average follow-up was 24 months (18–47 months) and all of the three-part fractures had good to very good functional results [constant score (14) 91% (range, 84–100)] without signs of AVN. With regard to four-part fractures, good radiographic results were achieved in valgus-impacted fractures with the exception of one patient, who developed partial necrosis of the humeral head. Patients with four-part fractures with lateral displacement, however, did not fare as well. One patient required prosthetic arthroplasty due to AVN, and another patient required revision to a prosthesis due to redisplacement of the fracture. The overall head necrosis rate of all patients with four-part fractures was 11%. The average constant score of all patients with four-part fractures and a preserved head (excluding the 2 failures) was 87% (range 79–100%).

Between 1995 and 1999, an additional 61 cases with three- (28) or four-part (33) fractures (most of them valgus impacted fractures) (19) were treated according to this technique and also confirmed the earlier results.

A Complications

No major complications occurred. There was no nerve palsy or infection. The only complications encountered were related to implant migration in older patients with osteoporotic bone. In two cases this was followed by fracture displacement, and reoperation with prosthetic replacement was necessary in one. No migration was seen when the Humerusblock (see below) was included in the treatment. In one case with a head-splitting fracture, the reduction could not be maintained even though the implants did not migrate. Open reconstruction was performed one week later.

B Pearls and Pitfalls

1 Fracture of the Greater Tuberosity

In cases of comminuted greater tuberosity fractures, screw fixation alone is usually not sufficient. In these cases it is recommended to fix the fragment by screws and additional transosseous sutures or with wire circlage, which can only be performed by open surgery.

Greater tuberosity reduction can be difficult to assess in the AP direction when viewing only on an AP view; however, there are several signs to look for to assure an adequate reduction: (1) the profile of the head has to show an anatomical appearance and (2) bone density must not show any abrupt change between head and fragment.

After the fragment has been temporarily fixed, the arm should be internally rotated maximally to assess the alignment on the posterior side. A persisting step-off between the tuberosity and the head confirms that the tuberosity is posteriorly displaced. Another option is to use the axillary view with the arm in 70° of abduction.

2 Fracture of the Lesser Tuberosity

The medial displacement of the fragment is caused by the pull of the subscapularis and is seen only in the axillary view. Reduction is performed with the arm abducted up to 70° and the central beam of the image intensifier positioned for an axillary view. The amount of displacement is shown by the height of the step-off in the articular surface caused by the medialized lesser tuberosity. Reduction is performed with the pointed hook retractor. With this instrument, the lesser tuberosity is engaged at the insertion of the tendon on the bone and is pulled laterally until the step-off of the articular surface has disappeared.

3 Fixation of the Fracture

Fixation of proximal humeral fractures with K-wires and screws is usually not a problem in young patients with good bone quality but may be problematic in elderly patients with osteoporosis. In these cases, K-wires may migrate and lead to loss of reduction and re-displacement. The following techniques are recommended to minimize these risks:

1. Use of threaded K-wires: The grip of the K-wires in the porotic bone is increased compared to regular K-wires but needs additional restrictions like stable arm fixation on the body for at least 10 days or 2 weeks.
2. Humerusblock (F/O group): This K-wire fixation device allows the insertion of two 2.2 mm K-wires via a guiding system and allows stable fixation of the wires by means of two locking screws in the block. As the

K-wires are fixed in the block and the cortex as well, rotational and axial stability of the head fragment is guaranteed. The K-wires allow setting of the head fragment along the K-wires, causing fast healing ("guided setting"). In patients with severe porotic bone, the tips of the K-wires are drilled through the subchondral bone to increase the grip in the bone. After 2–3 weeks, when movement exercises are started the K-wires are withdrawn below the subchondral bone under local anesthesia.

3. Postoperative movement: This depends on the bone quality and the number of fragments. Since percutaneous treatment causes little scar development, the arm can be immobilized for 2 weeks without any decrease in functional outcome. This is different than open treatment, in which early motion is often necessary to avoid significant loss of motion.

4 Axillary Nerve

The axillary nerve traverses the underside of the deltoid muscle at a distance of about 6 cm from the acromion; therefore, it may be in harm's way when screws are placed to secure the greater tuberosity. This can be avoided in one of the following three ways:

1. The stem of the axillary nerve forms terminal branches at the level of the lateral end of the acromion. Where the line of fracture permits, the screws should be placed from a slightly antero-lateral direction with the arm held in additional internal rotation.
2. If an approach in the area of the stem of the axillary nerve cannot be avoided, following skin incision, the trocar sheath with the blunt trocar should be advanced in a cranio-medial direction until bone is met and then slid down the bone caudally. The trocar sheath will thus keep the axillary nerve out of harm's way.
3. In the area of the axillary nerve, only screws without washer should be used in order to avoid entrapment of the nerve under the washer.

5 Age of Fracture

The time between accident and surgery is especially relevant in valgus impacted fractures. Although some cases were operated on successfully after 12 and 14 days, in general after 10 days separation of the impacted head from the shaft is difficult.

VI DISCUSSION

Percutaneous reduction of a fracture of the humeral head presupposes excellent understanding of the anatomy and the ability to visualize the fracture lines. The latter requires careful study of the radiographs, which must be available in at least two planes. We recommend Neer's trauma series and in some cases 3D CT scanning to better characterize the fracture pattern.

As with all percutaneous interventions to reduce articular fractures, the availability of residual soft tissue linking the various fragments is necessary in order to benefit from ligamentotaxis.

Three-part fractures with pronounced displacement in the subcapital area and avulsion of the greater tuberosity often involve internal malrotation of the humeral head plus angulation. There is often only a residual periosteal connection on the dorsal side, so that the humeral head is highly mobile. It is important to achieve reduction and fixation in the area of the humeral neck before seeking to reduce the tuberosity.

In the case of a severe humeral head fracture with four segments, a disruption of the greater and lesser tuberosity creates a situation in which the blood supply to the articular segment is maintained only via the periosteum extending to the medial part of the anatomical humeral neck (15,16). This periosteum has to be preserved at the time of surgery. The low rate of necrosis in an openly reconstructed fracture group, which we have operated and published in 1995, proves that surgical intervention did not further compromise the circulation when careful surgical techniques were used and the use of implants was kept to a minimum (17). The necrosis rate in valgus impacted humeral head fractures was about the same as it was with percutaneously treated cases (6,13,17). A comparison between the open and closed group of valgus impacted four-part fractures shows, however, that the functional results are slightly better with the percutaneous approach. Patients who were operated on using the percutaneous technique were able to return to work significantly earlier than those who underwent open surgery (on average 11 weeks in contrast to 14 weeks) (13). This may be due in part to decreased scar formation in the percutaneously treated patients. Consequently, postoperative functional improvement is obtained more quickly than with the open procedure.

Cancellous bone grafting after raising the impacted humeral head has not been employed with any patients using the closed procedure. Postoperative immobilization of the arm in adduction following percutanous reduction creates less pressure on the reduced head fragment than did the abduction plaster we earlier considered necessary following open surgery (17). Because closed treatment causes less scar development than open surgery, immobilization of the arm for up to 2 weeks postoperatively can be performed without the danger of stiffness.

One of the major problems in older patients with osteoporotic bone is migration of the K-wires. Therefore, the concern is not that a reduction can be obtained but that it may be difficult to hold. The introduction of the Humerusblock, which holds the K-wires, has dramatically decreased the likelihood of migration. Since we began using this implant, the average age of the patients treated percutaneously has increased to over 80 years.

Positioning for the patient is identical for both the percutaneous and open technique; if necessary, therefore, conversion to an open approach is quite simple in case percutaneous reconstruction has to be abandoned. Fractures with a questionable likelihood of success with the percutaneous technique can be treated with a percutaneous reconstruction first, and, if needed, conversion to an open reconstruction can be performed. However, even this should not be performed without having studied the type of fracture on good quality x-rays in three planes and perhaps an additional 3D CT scan.

VII CONCLUSIONS

Important features of the percutaneous technique are:

1.   A crucial factor for the success of percutaneous reconstruction is the presence of soft tissue bridging the various fragments, thus offering support in the form of ligamentotaxis.

2. In the case of three-part fractures and valgus impacted four-part fractures, the percutaneous reduction technique almost always produces good to very good functional results.
3. Because of the reduced availability of soft-tissue bridges between the fragments, four-part fractures with pronounced lateral displacement of the articular segment are clearly less suitable for the percutaneous technique than those without significant lateral displacement.
4. The necrosis rate is not increased by this technique.
5. In the absence of fracture exposure, adhesion within the surrounding gliding surface is reduced and the rehabilitation period is shorter than following open surgery.

REFERENCES

1. Mills EJ, Horne G. Fracture of the proximal humerus in adults. J Trauma 1985; 25:801–805.
2. Neer CS II. Displaced proximal humerus fractures, Part II. Treatment of three-part and four-part displacement. J Bone Joint Surg 1970; 52-A:1090–1103.
3. Stableforth PG. Four-part fractures of the neck of the humerus. J Bone Joint Surg 1984; 66B:104–108.
4. Svend-Hansen H. Displaced proximal humeral fractures. Acta Orthop Scand 1974; 45:359–364.
5. Jaberg H, Jakob RP. Trümmerfrakturen des proximalen Humerus. Orthopädie 1987; 16:320–335.
6. Jakob R, Miniaci A, Anson PS, Jaberg H, Osterwalder A, Ganz R. Four part valgus impacted fractures of the proximal humerus. *J Bone Joint* Surg 1991; 73 B(2):295–298.
7. Münst P, Kuner EH. Osteosynthesen bei dislozierten Humeruskopffrakturen. Orthopäde 1992; 21:121–130.
8. Böhler J. Percutane Osteosynthese mit dem Röntgenbildverstärker. Wien Klin Wochenschr 1962; 26:485–487.
9. Siebler G, Kuner EH. Late results after surgical treatment of proximal humerus fractures in adult persons. Unfallchirurgie 1985; 11:119–127.
10. Hausberger K, Resch H, Maurer H Blood supply of intraarticular fractures of the humeral head. An anatomical and biomechanical study. Lisbon: SECEC, 2000.
11. Müller ME, Allgöwer M, Schneider R, Willenegger H Manual der Osteosynthese. Heidelberg: Springer, 1992.
12. Neer CS II. Displaced proximal humerus fractures, Part I. Classification and evaluation. J Bone Joint Surg 1970; 52-A:1077–1089.
13. Resch H, Povacz P, Fröhlich H, Wainbacher M Percutaneous fixation of three- and four-part fractures of the proximal humerus. J Bone Joint Surg (Br) 1997; 79–13:295–300.
14. Constant CR, Murley AHG A clinical method of functional assessment of the shoulder. Clin Orthop 1987; 214:160–164.
15. Brooks CH, Revell WJ, Heatley FW. Vascularity of the humeral head after proximal humeral fractures—an anatomical study. J Bone Joint Surg (Br) 1993; 75-B:132–136.
16. Seggl W, Weiglein A. Die arterielle Blutversorgung des Oberarmkopfes und ihre prognostische Bedeutung bei Luxationen, Frakturen und Luxationsfrakturen des Oberarmkopfes. Acta Chirurg Austriaca 1991; 1:Suppl 92.
17. Resch H, Beck E, Bayley J. Reconstruction of valgus impacted humeral head fractures—indication, technique and long-term results. J Shoulder Elbow Surg 1995; 4:73–80.

3

Open Reduction and Internal Fixation of Greater and Lesser Tuberosity Fractures

MICHAEL Q. FREEHILL

University of Minnesota, Minneapolis, Minnesota, U.S.A.

WILLIAM N. LEVINE

Columbia University, College of Physicians and Surgeons, New York-Presbyterian Hospital, and Center for Shoulder, Elbow and Sports Medicine, New York, New York, U.S.A.

I PREOPERATIVE PLANNING

Appropriate decision-making in the treatment of displaced tuberosity fractures is based upon a thorough clinical examination and appropriate radiographic evaluation. A standard trauma series consisting of an anteroposterior and lateral view of the shoulder, obtained in the plane of the scapula, in addition to an axillary view will aid in determining the degree of fracture displacement (Fig. 1). If an axillary view is difficult to obtain due to the patient's pain, a Velpeau axillary may be obtained. This is taken with the patient hyperextending approximately 30° over the x-ray table with the beam passing vertically from a superior to inferior position in relation to the shoulder (1) (Fig. 2).

Further delineation of the fracture pattern can be obtained using various other imaging modalities, if necessary. A computed tomography (CT) scan can further evaluate the degree of fracture displacement, comminution, and integrity of the articular surface (Fig. 3). Some authors have advocated the use of a spiral CT with three-dimensional and multiplanar reconstructions, although this appears to be more useful when assessing complex three-part and four-part fractures (2) (Fig. 4). Magnetic resonance imaging (MRI) may also provide additional information regarding any associated soft tissue injuries, particularly those involving the rotator

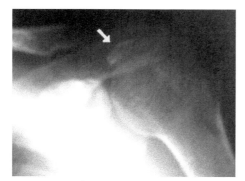

Figure 1 Plain AP radiograph demonstrating a comminuted greater tuberosity fracture with superior displacement of the fragment.

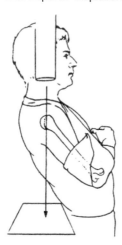

Figure 2 Proper positioning of the patient is demonstrated to obtain a Velpeau axillary view. (From Ref. 1.)

cuff, biceps tendon, or glenoid labrum. However, no studies have supported its routine use for evaluation of fractures. Since greater tuberosity and lesser tuberosity fractures often occur in conjunction with anterior and posterior dislocations, respectively, it is important to assess the vascular status of the patient prior to operative intervention. Vascular injury after a proximal humerus fracture is exceedingly rare, as only 16 cases of axillary arterial injury have been reported in the literature (2). Axillary arterial injuries are identified clinically with evidence of an expanding hematoma or an absent distal pulse. However, since distal pulses are reported to be palpable in 27% of patients with major arterial injuries proximally, any suspicion of a vascular injury necessitates a Doppler examination followed by arteriography if arterial compromise is suspected.

Numerous factors are taken into consideration when determining whether operative or nonoperative intervention is indicated. These include the patient's age, associated injuries, degree of fracture displacement, bone quality, arm dominance, and patient's preinjury activity level. When assessing a greater tuberosity fracture, the amount of displacement is the primary consideration. We recommend open

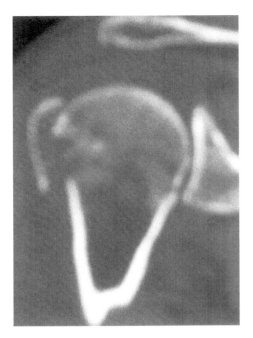

Figure 3 CT coronal image that demonstrates greater than 5 mm displacement of the tuberosity fragment.

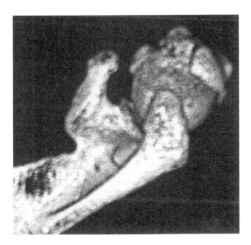

Figure 4 Axial CT reconstruction also demonstrates the posterior component of displacement.

reduction internal fixation for any fracture that is displaced more than 5 mm, especially when the displacement is superior (4–6). Displacement of this magnitude will frequently lead to impingement of the fragment below the acromion, thereby limiting the patient's functional return if allowed to heal in this position. In addition, posterior displacement may lead to further functional deficits, particularly in external rotation (5).

Isolated two-part lesser tuberosity fractures in the absence of an associated posterior dislocation are extremely rare. Frequently there is an associated nondisplaced surgical neck fracture, or these injuries can occur in conjunction with greater tuberosity fractures in young patients. When visualized, the fragment is often displaced medially, secondary to the pull of the subscapularis. If the fragment is large and includes a portion of the articular surface, it may impede internal rotation. This fracture configuration is often best treated by open reduction and internal fixation.

II OPERATIVE APPROACHES

Isolated greater tuberosity and lesser tuberosity fractures can be addressed through two basic surgical approaches. The greater tuberosity is most frequently approached through the superior transdeltoid approach due to the posterior-superior pull of the rotator cuff (Fig. 5). The skin incision is made within Langer's lines over the antero-lateral corner of the acromion, approximately 6–8 cm in length. The incision can be placed somewhat more posteriorly if necessary to address the more posteriorly displaced greater tuberosity fracture.

The approach for a two-part lesser tuberosity fracture involves the standard delto-pectoral approach. This will allow for mobilization of the lesser tuberosity and subscapularis.

Numerous fixation methods have been described in the literature (7–9). Both greater tuberosity and lesser tuberosity fractures have been fixed with AO interfragmentary screws; a tension band technique utilizing stainless wire or heavy suture material (#5 Ethibond or mersilene) has also been described. In general, screw fixation for both greater and lesser tuberosity fractures should be reserved for patients with good bone quality and with fractures consisting of a large, noncomminuted fragment.

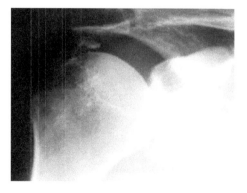

Figure 5 Preoperative right shoulder AP radiograph of a 52-year-old right-hand–dominant patient demonstrating superior displacement of the greater tuberosity.

III OUR PERSONAL APPROACH — GREATER TUBEROSITY FRACTURES

The authors prefer regional interscalene block for anesthesia. This provides a safe, effective means of anesthesia during the procedure and significant pain relief for the patient in the early postoperative period. The patient is then placed in the high beach chair position in a well-padded headrest. All bony prominences must be adequately padded, as the patient is brought to the edge of the operating table. This positioning allows for the injured arm to be brought into extension, which ultimately facilitates exposure of the proximal humerus. The sterile preparation should include the entire shoulder, lateral neck, axilla, chest wall, and ipsilateral arm to the level of the wrist. The arm is draped free to allow for adequate positioning throughout the procedure. Broad-spectrum intravenous antibiotics are administered prior to incision.

The isolated greater tuberosity fracture is exposed through the superior deltoid approach (Fig. 6A). After the skin incision is made within Langer's lines along the anterolateral aspect of the acromion, the deltoid is then split off the acromion approximately 3–4 cm (Fig. 6B). It is important not to violate the deltoid origin during exposure. If necessary, the deltoid split can be made more posteriorly off the lateral edge of the acromion to allow for adequate visualization of the posterior displaced greater tuberosity fracture. The deltoid split is completed using needle tip electrocautery, thereby minimizing trauma to the deltoid muscle. An antipropagation

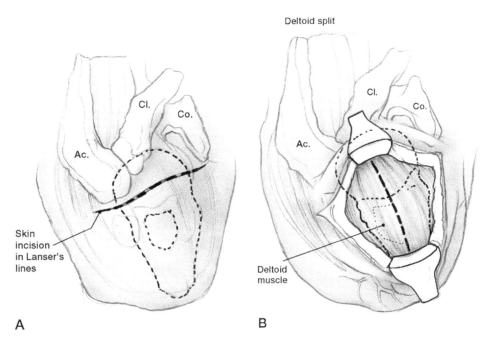

Figure 6 (A) Anterosuperior approach for exposure of the greater tuberosity fragment. The skin incision should be made within Langer's lines for a good cosmetic appearance. (B) Deltoid split from the anterolateral corner of the acromion. The split can be placed more posterior if required. The transdeltoid approach should not proceed further than 3–4 cm from the lateral acromion to avoid iatrogenic injury to the axillary nerve. Ac. = Acromion; Cl. = clavicle; Co. = coracoid.

suture is placed at the distal extent of the deltoid split to prevent possible injury to the circumflex branch of the axillary nerve. The muscle is then retracted anteriorly and posteriorly to allow for lysis of subacromial adhesions. All hemorrhagic bursa and inflamed soft tissue should be adequately excised to allow for visualization of the bony edges of the displaced fragment. Internal rotation of the arm facilitates exposure of the displaced greater tuberosity. Gentle downward traction on the arm may also increase the subacromial space to improve exposure. Continuous and excessive traction, however, should be avoided in order to prevent neurological injury.

Once the fracture bed and greater tuberosity are identified and all hematoma and soft tissue remnants are cleared from the region, the greater tuberosity can be mobilized. Heavy #5 nonabsorbable sutures are placed at the bone-tendon junction to allow for appropriate reduction for the superiorly and posteriorly displaced fragment (Fig. 7). It is important to avoid placing the sutures through the greater tuberosity, as the rotator cuff tendon–bone junction is often stronger than the

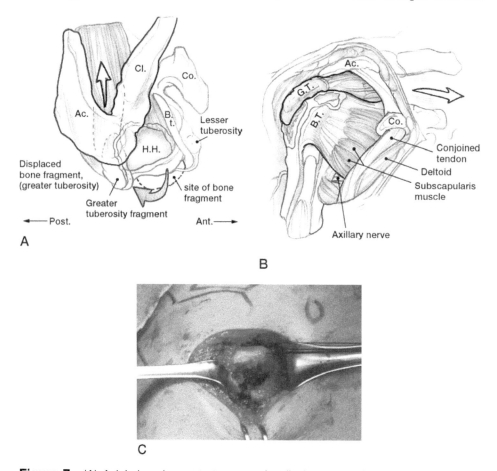

Figure 7 (A) Axial view demonstrates posterior displacement of the greater tuberosity fragment. (B) AP view demonstrates superior displacement of the greater tuberosity fragment into the subacromial space. (C) Intraoperative photo of right shoulder demonstrating mobilized greater tuberosity and fracture bed. Ac. = Acromion, B.T. = biceps tendon, Cl. = clavicle, Co. = Coracoid, G.T. = greater tuberosity, H.H. = humeral head.

ostoeporotic bone of the tuberosity. After mobilization of the fragment, the remaining portion of the rotator cuff is identified for any additional injury. These fractures are frequently found to have tears involving the rotator interval anteriorly or between the supraspinatus and infraspinatus, depending on the location of the fracture. If repair of the rotator interval or associated rotator cuff tear is to be undertaken, sutures should be placed in an interrupted tendon-to-tendon fashion prior to final reduction of the fracture, as this will facilitate the repair of the soft tissue injury.

Attention is turned to the greater tuberosity fragment and fracture bed. The fragment may require fashioning with a rongeur to allow for adequate reduction into the fracture bed and to prevent any impingement lesion from occurring secondary to a prominent portion of the greater tuberosity. Transosseous tunnels are created in the region of the fracture bed allowing for a 1 cm cortical bridge between the fracture bed and the intact proximal humerus (Fig. 8A). Multiple #5 nonabsorbable sutures

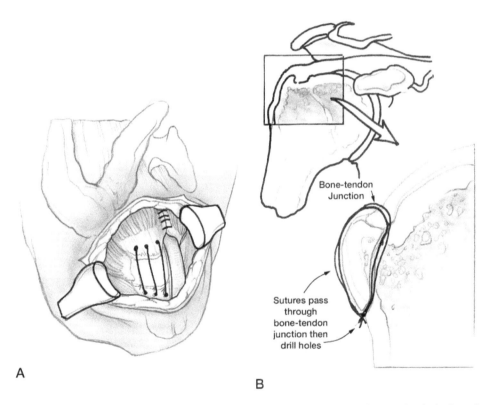

A

B

Figure 8 (A) Axial view demonstrating transosseous sutures in the proximal shaft and tuberosity fragment prior to anatomical reduction. (B) Concept of suture placement at the bone-tendon junction of the tuberosity. (C) Intraoperative photo of right shoulder demonstrating sutures at bone-tendon junction with anatomical reduction of tuberosity. (D) Reduction of the fragment is demonstrated with augmentation of the tuberosity to shaft fixation utilizing horizontal tuberosity-to-tuberosity sutures. The repair is then secured with closure of the lateral aspect of the rotator interval. (E) Intraoperative photo of right shoulder showing final suture fixation with associated rotator interval closure. (F) Final postoperative AP radiograph (6 months) with anatomical restoration of the displaced greater tuberosity. The patient had regained full range of motion and strength and had no symptoms.

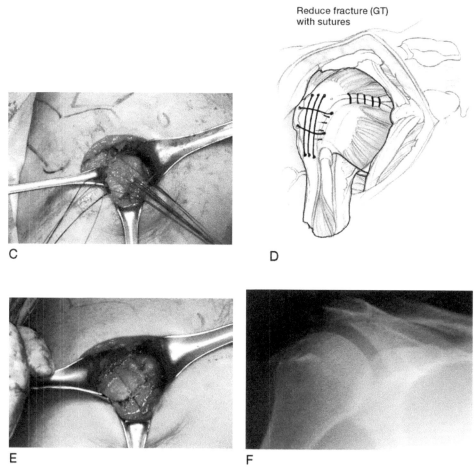

Figure 8 Continued.

are placed through the drill holes and into the fracture fragment at the bone-tendon junction (Fig. 8B,C). The greater tuberosity is then reduced into place and the sutures tied in serial fashion. An associated rotator interval closure and/or rotator cuff repair is then performed using several #0 nonabsorbable sutures (Fig. 8D,E). This is a vital part of the repair, as this will effectively reduce the forces across the fracture site. In addition, this will help further stabilize the fracture fragment. The arm is then taken through a range of motion to check for stability and also to assess for any persistent impingement during elevation or external rotation. This range-of-motion testing will also help guide the surgeon in recommending postoperative physical therapy. Radiographs should confirm anatomical restoration of the greater tuberosity postoperatively (Fig. 8F).

IV OUR PERSONAL APPROACH — LESSER TUBEROSITY FRACTURES

The isolated lesser tuberosity fracture is extremely rare, and the authors have never treated such an injury. However, displaced lesser tuberosity fractures can occur in younger patients following high-energy injuries to the proximal humerus (Fig. 9A, B). This injury can be approached through a deltopectoral incision. The deltopectoral interval is identified and split, retracting the cephalic vein laterally. The lateral edge of the conjoined tendon and the coracoid are visualized. The clavipectoral fascia is incised and retracted with the deltoid. The hemorrhagic bursa and hematoma is subsequently excised. The lesser tuberosity fragment is identified and mobilization is initiated. Several #2 or #5 nonabsorbable sutures are placed at the bone-tendon junction between the subscapularis and the lesser tuberosity. To allow for adequate mobilization, the rotator interval may require further division if not already completed by the fracture. In addition, all adjacent subcoracoid adhesions should be released. Furthermore, the axillary nerve should be identified and protected throughout the entire procedure, particularly when mobilizing a fragment that may be several weeks old. Also, the long head of the biceps may be dislocated medially or its presence may inhibit appropriate visualization and/or reduction, thus requiring tenotomy and subsequent tenodesis.

After adequate mobilization, the lesser tuberosity and fracture bed are prepared for reduction (Fig. 10A,B). The choice of fixation is chosen based on the size of the fragment, the quality of the bone, and the presence or absence of comminution. For younger patients with good bone, little comminution, and a single large fragment, screw fixation may be appropriate. However, if there is any uncertainty with the quality of the repair, multiple heavy suture fixation should be used either in addition to or in place of screw fixation. The fragment may need to be fashioned with a rongeur to allow for appropriate and secure placement into the fracture bed. Transosseous tunnels are created in the region of the proximal humerus, leaving a 1 cm cortical bridge between the fracture bed and the drill holes. At this time, the intra-articular portion of the biceps is released. A tenodesis is

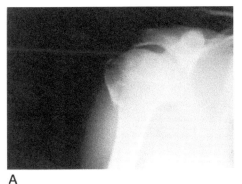
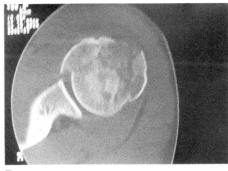

A   B

Figure 9 (A) AP x-ray of right shoulder of 31-year-old patient with displaced lesser tuberosity and minimally displaced greater tuberosity fractures. (B) CT scan demonstrating medial displacement of lesser tuberosity fracture (note attached bicipital groove with lesser tuberosity).

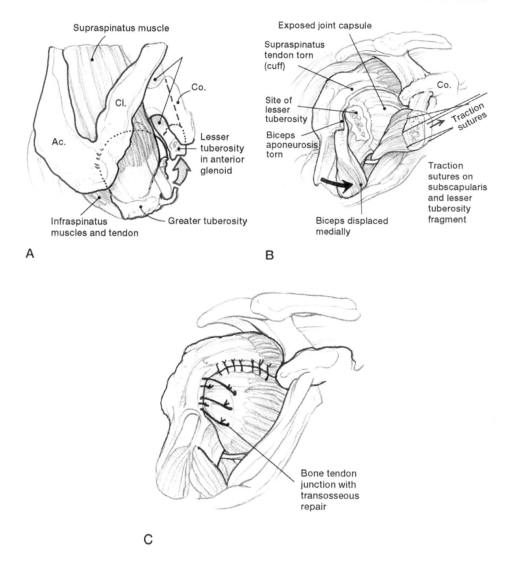

Figure 10 (A) Axial view demonstrating medial displacement of the lesser tuberosity fragment and disruption of the medial wall of the biceps groove. (B) Mobilization of the fragment with traction sutures and release of all subcoracoid and intra-articular-based adhesions. The biceps is prepared for tenodesis if dislocated or subluxed medially. (C) Transosseous sutures passed through the tendon-bone junction are secured in serial fashion with augmentation of the repair through closure of the lateral aspect of the rotator interval. Ac. = Acromion; Cl. = clavicle; Co. = coracoid.

performed using transosseous sutures or suture anchors in the region of the biceps groove. The biceps groove, if present to any extent, is prepared to a punctate, bleeding surface. Transosseous sutures are then placed in an interrupted fashion through the biceps proximally and secured in an interrupted fashion. Attention is then turned to the lesser tuberosity. Multiple #5 nonabsorbable sutures are placed through the transosseous tunnels and into the bone-tendon junction of the lesser tuberosity and subscapularis. The sutures should be placed along an equal distribution of the tuberosity extending superiorly to inferiorly to allow for an adequate reduction of the fragment. The sutures are tied in sequential fashion from superior to inferior. The lateral aspect of the rotator interval is reapproximated using #0 nonabsorbable sutures (Fig. 10C). The area is copiously irrigated, and the shoulder is taken through full range of motion to assess for stability of the fracture fragment. It is important to note the extent of external rotation that is achieved while the patient is on the operating table, as this will direct the range of motion recommended at the time of physical therapy. After examination, the deltopectoral interval is loosely approximated with #0 nonabsorbable sutures. The subcutaneous tissue and skin are then closed in layers using an absorbable suture, followed by application of steri-strips. The patient is placed in a sling, and physical therapy is initiated on the first postoperative day. Postoperative radiographs should confirm anatomical reduction and in this case proper screw positioning (Fig. 11).

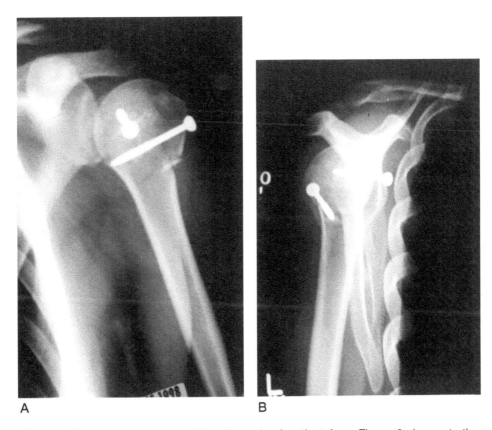

A   B

Figure 11 (A) Postoperative AP radiograph of patient from Figure 9 demonstrating anatomical restoration of the proximal humerus with 4.5 mm screw fixation of lesser and greater tuberosities. (B) Postoperative scapular lateral radiograph of same patient demonstrating anatomical restoration of the proximal humerus with appropriate screw placement.

V PEARLS AND PITFALLS

A. Greater Tuberosity
  1. Avoid using screws in osteoporotic bone.
  2. Avoid using screws when multiple fracture lines are present (along the facets).
  3. Use the bone-tendon junction to your advantage in older, osteopenic patients by using transosseous tunnels and heavy nonabsorbable sutures.
  4. Always image the shoulder with 90° orthogonal views to assure anatomic reduction.
  5. Anterosuperior approach preferred in majority of cases.

B. Lesser Tuberosity
  1. Much rarer injury in isolation.
  2. May be amenable to screw fixation if bone is of good quality (usually one large piece, as opposed to greater tuberosity which may fracture along facet lines).
  3. Use the rotator interval to your advantage (open it up) to improve visualization and anatomic reduction and fixation.
  4. Deltopectoral approach is preferred in all cases.

VI REHABILITATION

The authors recommend the use of the three-phase system, originally described by Hughes and Neer (8). The initial range of motion that will be allowed is determined at the time of surgery. The surgeon must assess the stability of the fixation in order to define the amount of forward elevation and external rotation. Ultimately, the rehabilitation program is individualized based on the stability of the fracture fixation and the patient's ability to cooperate during therapy. In general, a sling is used for protection for the first 6 weeks. During this interval, the patient may remove the sling to perform the therapy program. The basic program focuses on active range of motion of the elbow, wrist, and hand with early passive range of motion to the shoulder. The authors typically begin passive range of motion on the first postoperative day. Elevation is performed in the plane of the scapula, as assisted by the surgeon or therapist. The patient will be instructed in pendulum exercises in addition to supine passive external rotation with a cane within the defined range of motion limits. This program is continued for approximately 6 weeks until evidence of tuberosity healing is apparent on radiographs. We discourage the use of pulleys in the early postoperative period since active firing of muscles does occur and can lead to pull-off of the repaired tuberosity.

   Subsequently, assisted active elevation and external rotation with isometric strengthening of the rotator cuff and deltoid are begun approximately 6–8 weeks after the operation. As range of motion and strength progresses, the patient is encouraged to use the involved upper extremity for activities of daily living as tolerated. Gentle pain-free stretching is advocated during this phase to ensure that motion is maintained, while focusing on primarily glenohumeral and scapulothoracic motion. Approximately 3 months after operative intervention, more aggressive stretching and resistance-type strengthening exercises are initiated. As the patient regains nearly full motion, progressive resistance training utilizing theraband or light free weights ranging from 1–3 lb. are used. It is important to communicate to the patient during this rehabilitation period that it may take 12–18 months to achieve maximum benefits. However, most of the recovery often occurs within the first 6–9 months.

It is important to modify the rehabilitation program as healing progresses. The authors recommend obtaining radiographs approximately 2 weeks following surgery to confirm maintenance of appropriate position of the tuberosities. Additional radiographs should be obtained at 6 weeks postoperatively, prior to advancing to a more active rehabilitation program. Overall, strict adherence to a physician-guided rehabilitation program will help ensure the best possibility for a satisfactory functional outcome.

REFERENCES

1. Post M, Bigliani LU, Flatow EL, Pollock RG. The Shoulder. Baltimore, MD: Williams and Wilkins. 1998, p. 47.
2. Jurik AG, Albrechtsen J. The use of computed tomography with two- and three-dimensional reconstructions in the diagnosis of three- and four- part fractures of the proximal humerus. Clin Radiol 1994; 49:800–804.
3. Zuckerman JD, Checroun AJ. Fractures of the proximal humerus: diagnosis and management. In: Iannotti JP, Williams GR, eds. Disorders of the Shoulder: Diagnosis and Management. Philadelphia: Lippincott Williams and Wilkins, 1999:639–685.
4. McLaughlin HL. Posterior dislocation of the shoulder. J Bone Joint Surg 1952; 34A:584–590.
5. Flatow EL, Cuomo F, Maday MG, et al. Open reduction and internal fixation of two-part displaced fractures of the greater tuberosity of the proximal part of the humerus. J Bone Joint Surg 1991; 73A:1213–1218.
6. Bono CM, Renard R, Levine RG, Levy AS. Effect of displacement of fractures of the greater tuberosity on the mechanics of the shoulder. J Bone Joint Surg 2001; 83A:1056–1062.
7. Bigliani LU. Treatment of two- and three- part Fractures of the proximal humerus. Am Acad Orthop Surg Instruct Course Lect 1989; 39:231–244.
8. Hawkins RJ, Kiefer GN. Internal fixation techniques for proximal humerus fractures. Clin Orthop 1987; 223:77–85.
9. Jaberg H, Warner JP, Jakob RP. Percutaneous stabilization of unstable fractures of the humerus. J Bone Joint Surg 1992; 74A:508–515.
10. Hughes M, Neer CS. Glenohumeral joint replacement and post-operative rehabilitation. Phys Ther 1975; 55:850–858.

4

Open Reduction and Internal Fixation of Surgical Neck Fractures

ARIANE GERBER

Campus Virchow-Klinikum, Humboldt University, Berlin, Germany

JON J. P. WARNER

Massachusetts General Hospital and Brigham & Women's Hospital, Boston, Massachusetts, U.S.A.

I INTRODUCTION

Surgical neck fractures account for approximately 60–65% of all proximal humeral fractures in adults. Nearly 80% are minimally displaced and can be treated nonoperatively. Stable impacted, but severely angulated fractures (10% of all surgical neck fractures) with an intact posterior periosteal sleeve, as well as displaced surgical neck fractures with or without metaphyseal comminution (10% of all surgical neck fractures) are usually treated operatively in the absence of medical contraindications. Indeed, nonoperative management of displaced (unstable or impacted) fractures does not consistently lead to good clinical outcomes. In a recent series of 56 surgical neck fractures treated nonoperatively, Chun et al. reported that only 31 patients (55%) had an excellent or good result at a mean follow-up of 6.6 years (5). The mean forward flexion of the overall series was 107°. Another series reported 15% poor or unsatisfactory long-term results after nonoperatively treated surgical neck fractures (6). Deformity and stiffness due to immobilization are the most common negative sequelae of such treatment (6). Many different surgical procedures have been proposed to stabilize surgical neck fractures, including minimally invasive fixation such as percutaneous pinning (10–12), external fixation (14), plate fixation (9), or intramedullary stabilization (2,15).

As in all displaced proximal humeral fractures, the appropriate therapeutic approach is based on a precise evaluation of the fracture pattern, estimation of the bone quality, consideration of specific problems such as avascular necrosis or nonunion, and appreciation of patient's compliance.

A   Surgical Neck Fractures and Avascular Necrosis

In surgical neck fractures the epiphyseal fragment usually remains vascularized since the ascending branch of the anterior circumflex artery and the vascular anastomoses from the posterior circumflex artery and from the joint capsule are intact (7). Rarely, a lesion of the axillary artery may occur where it is tethered to the humerus by the anterior and posterior humeral circumflex arteries. On occasion this can lead to avascular necrosis of the humeral articular fragment (20). Furthermore, the blood supply to the proximal fragment and the articular fragment, respectively, can be compromised through extensive dissection and/or plate fixation (18).

B   Surgical Neck Fractures and Nonunion

Although the prevalence of nonunion following proximal humeral fractures is not known, the surgical neck is the most frequent location for this complication. Neer reported 23% nonunions at the surgical neck in his series (16), and Jupiter and Mullaji described eight nonunions after displaced surgical neck fractures in a series of nine cases (13). The bone quality of the distal fragment and its mobility due to the lack of capsular attachment to the unopposed deforming force of the pectoralis major muscle may be responsible for the higher nonunion rate found at this level. Severe initial displacement of the fracture increases the mobility between the fragments accounting for the higher nonunion rate seen following fracture-dislocation. Other factors, more related to the chosen treatment modalities, such as inadequate immobilization, poor reduction due to tissue interposition, distraction, and insufficient fixation, have been implicated as well.

C   Surgical Neck Fractures and Malunion

Malunion at the surgical neck is better tolerated than malunion between the tuberosities and the humeral head (8). However, varus malunion of the surgical neck has been recognized as a cause of impingement (16). The amount of initial acceptable displacement has not been clearly determined, but simple acromioplasty has been reported to alleviate the symptoms (16). Extension malunion may also occur after nonoperative treatment of impacted surgical neck fractures. Typically, these fractures are angulated with the apex positioned anteriorly. Neer recommended that the deformity be accepted with the understanding that flexion and abduction may be lost in direct proportion to fracture angulation (16).

D   Surgical Neck and Associated Injuries

Due to their location, the neurovascular structures are at risk in surgical neck fractures; injury may occur from direct contact with the medially displaced distal fragment or from traction injuries. Brachial plexus injuries are also at great risk following fracture-dislocations. An electromyographic analysis has demonstrated that the incidence of axillary nerve lesions with glenohumeral dislocation and surgical neck fractures is 20–30%. Most of the lesions are neurapraxias and recover within months (1). However if re-innervation does not occur within 3–6 months, exploration and possible nerve repair should be performed early (3). Rupture, thrombus formation, and pseudoaneurysms of the axillary artery have been described with surgical neck fractures. Vascular injuries are usually associated with severe medial displacement of the distal fragment. If vascular reconstruction is indicated, stable fixation of the fracture should be performed prior vascular repair.

II PREOPERATIVE PLANNING

A Clinical Evaluation

Although detailed clinical evaluation of the shoulder in the presence of an acute fracture is difficult due to pain, a complete physical examination of the patient should be performed. A nerve injury should be excluded through meticulous neurological examination. Vascular injuries can present with only subtle clinical signs like swelling. Although the injured extremity can remain partially perfused through collateral circulation, the diagnosis should be confirmed and the indication for reconstruction established with an angiogram. This can avoid late complications such as Volkman's ischemic contracture. A vascular injury should be suspected in the presence of a severely displaced fracture or if a nerve injury is present. In severe trauma, fractures of the ipsilateral extremity, the cervical spine, or the chest wall may occur in addition to the proximal humeral fracture.

B Radiographic Evaluation

Conventional radiographic evaluation is essential for assessment of fracture configuration, choice of the adequate treatment, and preoperative planning. Surgical neck fractures can be diagnosed and classified with a conventional anteroposterior view, an axillary view, and a scapular lateral view of the injured shoulder. The anteroposterior view gives information about the amount of medial displacement of the distal fragment and the extent of metaphyseal comminution of the fracture. The axillary view is essential to evaluate the presence of an associated glenohumeral dislocation and to determine the amount of anterior angulation.

C Indication

Reducible angulated or displaced fractures without metaphyseal comminution represent the optimal indication for closed reduction and percutaneous pinning in reliable patients with good bone quality (see Chap. 2).

Some fractures cannot be reduced by closed techniques due to soft tissue entrapment. Either the biceps tendon or the pectoralis major tendon may be interposed in the facture (16). In severely displaced fractures, the distal fragment can be entrapped in the deltoid muscle, and in some cases open reduction is required to avoid iatrogenic injury due to the manipulation. The method of fixation depends on the bone quality and the surgeon's preference.

In the elderly patient with poor bone quality, initial stabilization with pins is probably not appropriate (8). Poor compliance and understanding during the postoperative phase in this group of patients often result in complications, such as pin loosening, secondary displacement or even nonunion. For these reasons, we prefer to perform open reduction and stable internal fixation, allowing immediate postoperative mobilization in the elderly patient in the absence of medical contraindications. In some fractures suture fixation can lead to stable fixation.

The combination of Ender nails with interfragmentary sutures improves the torsional load by a factor of 1.5 compared to sutures alone and may be required in certain fractures (2). Plate fixation, preferably with a blade plate, is another option that is recommended to achieve stable fixation.

Closed reduction and percutaneous pinning is not indicated in fractures with metaphyseal comminution. If the medial humeral neck of the proximal fragment cannot be reduced in a stable configuration over the distal diaphysis, pinning does not provide enough stability, and secondary displacement with or without nonunion may occur. If the comminution is limited to a large medial fragment, then open reduction and fixation of the fragment with screws will transform the fracture into a simple surgical neck fracture, which can then be further stabilized with percutaneous pinning. This is only an option in patients with good bone quality. If the medial fragment is too small to be fixed separately, in the presence of extensive comminution or poor bone quality, external fixation, intramedullary stabilization, or plate fixation are possible options.

In the presence of an associated injury requiring an open approach like a vascular lesion, stable fixation of the fracture is mandatory prior to vascular repair. In patients with multiple injuries, stable fixation allowing immediate postoperative mobilization may be an advantage in the rehabilitation phase. In open fractures requiring debridement, open reduction and internal or external fixation is a reasonable option.

III OPERATIVE APPROACHES

A Open Reduction, Minimal Invasive Fixation

Limited exposure and minimally invasive fixation have been proposed to limit additional vascular damage and decrease the risk of avascular necrosis (12). If a simple displaced surgical neck fracture requires open reduction, minimally invasive fixation can be achieved with percutaneous pinning provided the bone quality is adequate (see Chap. 2). In the case of medial comminution, the metaphyseal fragment(s) can be fixed with screws to transform the fracture into a simple surgical neck fracture. Pinning can then be added to fix the proximal fragment to the distal reconstructed diaphysis (Fig. 1).

In simple surgical neck fractures, impaction of the diaphyseal fragment in the cancellous neck region of the proximal fragment and fixation with heavy nonabsorbable sutures leads to stable fixation. The limited amount of shortening (0.5–1 cm) rarely limits function (Fig. 2).

B Open Reduction, Intramedullary Fixation

Intramedullary devices may be used after open reduction of surgical neck fractures. One biomechanical study has suggested their superior biomechanical properties, compared to pin fixation (19). However, a significant disadvantage of intramedullary nails is the necessity to violate the rotator cuff. Standard humeral rods are difficult to use in surgical neck fractures because the proximal fragment is short and therefore difficult to stabilize. Rods allowing interlocking to control the proximal fragment are available, but sufficient purchase of the screws is not always provided, especially if the bone quality is poor. Intramedullary Enders nail(s) combined with inter-

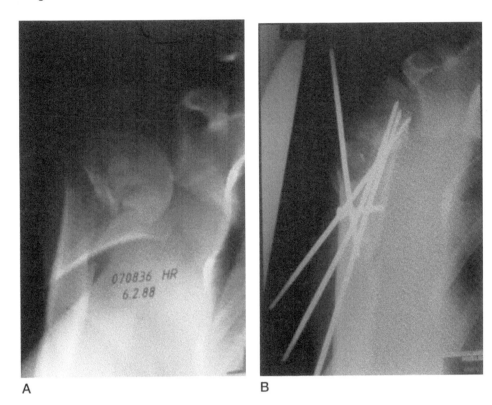

A B

Figure 1 (A) Surgical neck fracture with metaphyseal comminution. (B) The fragment is large enough and the bone quality is good, however, so that it can be transformed into a simple surgical neck fracture through open reduction and minimal internal fixation. (C and D) Radiographic and clinical results 4 months after the procedure.

fragmentary sutures provides excellent fixation (2). The technique is demanding, however, and optimal nail and suture placement is mandatory to avoid nonunion (Fig. 3). Like other nail systems, an approach through the rotator cuff is necessary (however, the incision is quite small and easily repaired following insertion).

C Open Reduction, Plate Fixation

Plate fixation to treat proximal humeral fractures has been shown to increase the rate of avascular necrosis (18). Extensive approach and plate placement can compromise the blood supply of the articular fragment. This may be more likely when broad implants like T-plates are used. Furthermore, conventional plates are not appropriate to achieve indirect reduction of proximal humeral fractures, especially when the bone quality is poor. Consequently, additional dissection is necessary to reduce and temporarily hold the fracture. Finally, the purchase of the screws in the proximal fragment may be poor, which limits postoperative rehabilitation.

Blade plate fixation for surgical neck fractures has been proposed by Bosworth (4) and used successfully by others (17). Although the mechanical properties of this implant have been shown to be comparable with the AO T-plate (17), this fixation

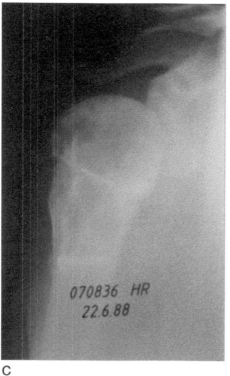

070836 HR
22.6.88

C

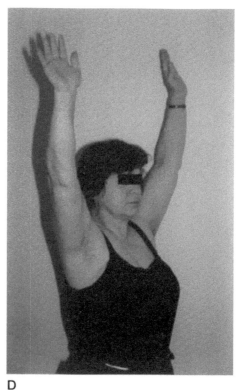

D

Figure 1 Continued.

technique has not gained wide popularity, probably due to the poor reputation of plate fixation for proximal humerus fractures. Recently, Jupiter designed a humeral blade plate for nonunion fixation of the surgical neck and achieved union in eight of nine nonunions (13). Only one series using this implant to treat acute fractures has been published (9). In this series, 42 elderly patients with three- and four-part fractures were treated with blade plate fixation. Union was achieved in an acceptable position in all patients, and avascular necrosis occurred in only two cases.

IV PERSONAL APPROACH: BLADE PLATE FIXATION

A Biological and Biomechanical Considerations

The 3.5 version of the AO humeral blade plate is a narrow plate, which can be placed on the lateral side of the bicipital groove without compromising the ascending branch of the anterior circumflex artery (Fig. 4). The stability of the blade in the humeral head is sufficient to allow for manipulation of the proximal fragment and indirect reduction, even if the bone quality is poor. The shortest blade (30 mm) can be introduced below the insertion of the rotator cuff on the greater tuberosity without perforation of the joint, which allows the fixation of very proximal surgical neck fractures (Fig. 5). The implant is rigid enough to stabilize fractures with comminution without additional fixation of the medial calcar region (bridging plate).

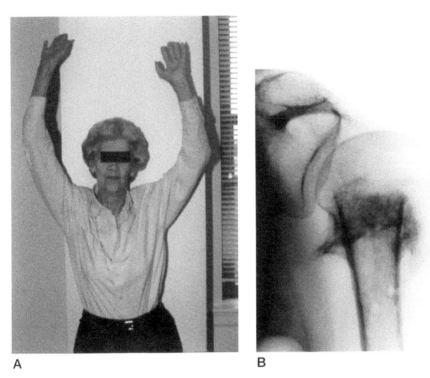

A   B

Figure 2   Result after simple suture fixation. The limited shortening does not influence function.

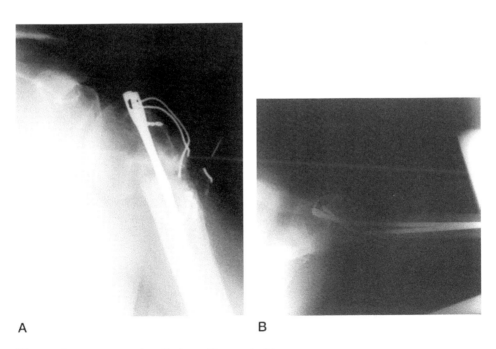

A   B

Figure 3   Nonunion after Ender nailing and wiring.

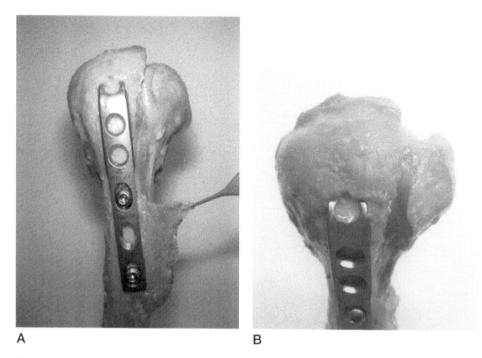

A   B

Figure 4 Cadaveric model (right humerus) showing optimal placement of the AO-blade plate. The plate is placed lateral to the bicipital groove and the pectoralis major tendon.

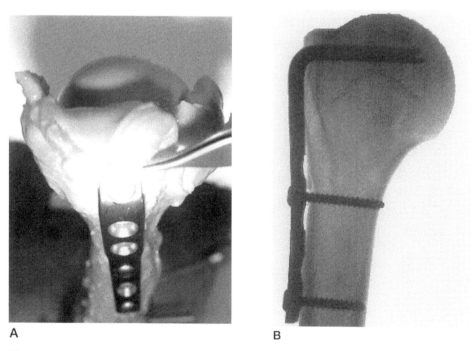

A   B

Figure 5 The blade can be placed safely in the humeral head even if introduced very proximally, below the insertion of the rotator cuff.

Finally, the LC-DCP design of the plate allows for interfragmentary compression if required.

B Surgical Technique

Preoperative planning is critical if open reduction and internal fixation with a humeral blade place is to be considered. (Fig. 6).

The patient is positioned on the operating table in the beach chair position. A long beanbag is used to securely position the patient so that fluoroscopic images can be obtained during the procedure. Prior to sterilely preparing and draping the upper extremity, a biplanar fluoroscopy C-arm unit is positioned so that both an anteroposterior and axillary view can be obtained during the procedure.

A deltopectoral approach is used, exposing exclusively the subdeltoid space on the lateral side of the bicipital grove and the insertion of the pectoralis major tendon (Figs. 7C and 8A). The insertion of the deltoid is elevated subperiosteally if a longer plate is used. The pectoralis major tendon remains intact. The planes between the pectoralis major muscle and the conjoined tendon and the conjoined tendon and the subscapularis muscle are not dissected. A 2.5 mm threaded blade plate K-wire is introduced in the proximal fragment, at least 1.5 cm above the fracture level and taking the version and the amount of displacement into consideration. The position of the wire is confirmed in the AP and axillary views. Once the K-wire is in adequate position, a cannulated blade plate (usually 30 mm blade) is introduced (attached to the plate holder) into the humeral head over the guide wire. In young patients with good bone quality, the introduction of the plate can be facilitated by opening the cortex with a 2.5 mm drill. The plate holder is used to reduce the proximal fragment (Fig. 9). In this position, the localization of the blade in the humeral head is confirmed fluoroscopically before fixation. A small Verbrugge clamp is used to fix the plate temporarily to the distal fragment. If adequate reduction is achieved the plate is fixed in the distal fragment with screws. If the purchase of the cortical screws is suboptimal, 4.0 mm cancellous screws can be used in the same hole, usually with better fixation (Fig. 7F,G). Cement augmentation is an alternative, but is rarely required. For simple fractures, compression can be achieved with the use of either eccentric screws or plate tensioning device.

A screw placed in the hole of the plate's bend is introduced from a lateral-proximal to medial-distal direction. Even if the distal fragment cannot be reached, this screw should be used to enhance stability of the blade in the proximal fragment (Figs. 7F and 8B).

In severely comminuted fractures, a distractor can be used to reduce and stabilize the fracture. This can significantly facilitate the proper placement of the plate without additional dissection (Fig. 8A).

If this implant is used to fix the surgical neck component of a three-part fracture, the holes of the plate can be used to attach the sutures used for tuberosity fixation (Fig. 7D,E).

V PEARLS AND PITFALLS

1. Avoid the temptation to use percutaneous pinning techniques in elderly patients or in patients with poor bone quality.

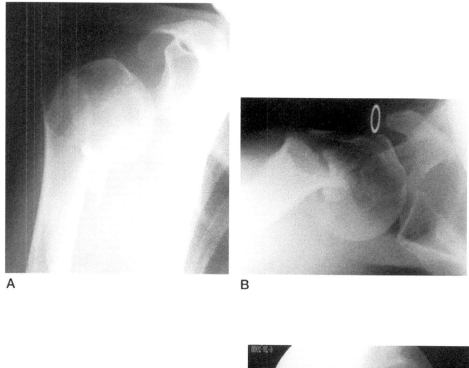

A   B

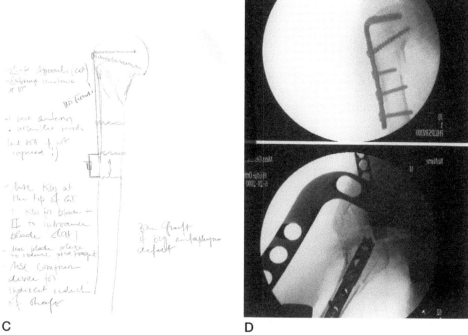

C   D

Figure 6   (A and B) Example of a fracture with medial metaphyseal comminution and severe anterior angulation. (C) Preoperative planning helps to define the plate dimensions and its optimal placement. The plan was to reduce the fracture with the plate-tensioning device used as distractor. (D) Postoperative radiographic results.

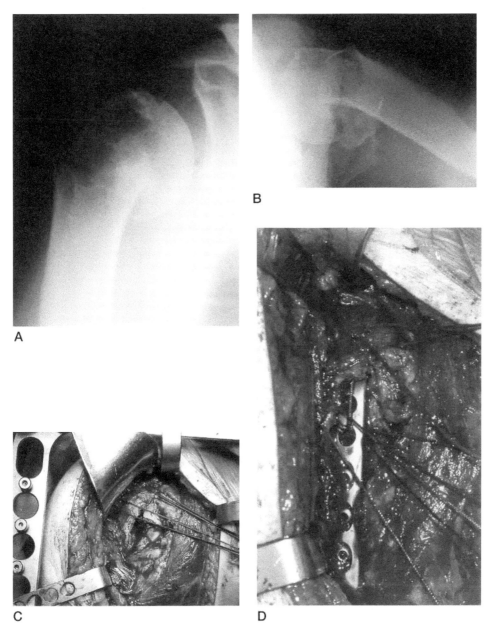

Figure 7   AP (A) and axillary (B) of a displaced surgical neck fracture component of a 3-part greater tuberosity fracture in an elderly patient. (C) Only the subdeltoid plane is exposed leaving the medial soft tissue sleeve intact. Heavy nonabsorbable sutures have been used to mobilize the greater tuberosity. (D and E) The surgical neck component is reduced and stabilized with a blade plate and the plate is used to fix the suture, securing the greater tuberosity. No dissection of the medial tissue was required to stabilize the fracture. (F and G) Postoperative radiographs. Note that cancellous 4.0 screws were used to enhance purchase in the shaft. The oblique screw in the blade plate bend enhances stability of the blade in the proximal fragment.

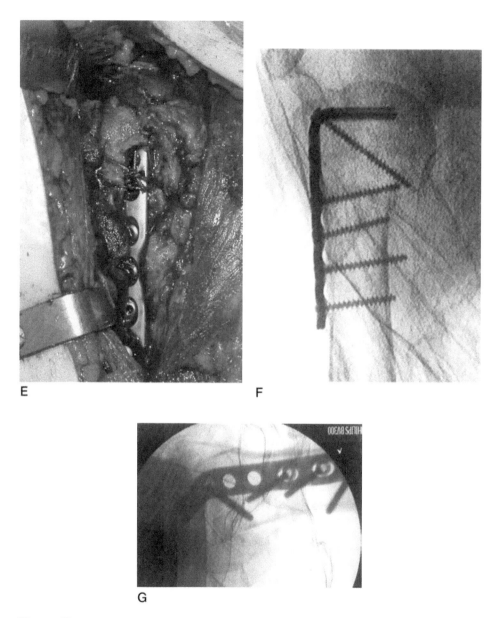

E

F

G

Figure 7 Continued.

2. The blade plate offers excellent initial stability for intraoperative manipulation of the fragments and for postoperative management of the patient.
3. Placement of the blade plate on the lateral side of the bicipital groove avoids the ascending branch of the anterior circumflex artery.
4. Place a screw in the plate's bend from a lateral-proximal to medial-distal direction to enhance stability of the blade in the proximal fragment.

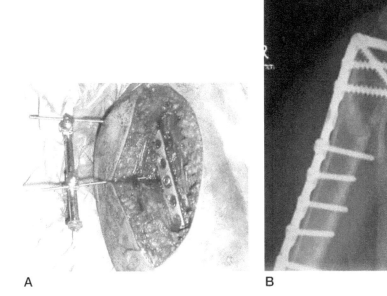

Figure 8   (A) The distractor is used to reduce the fracture. Only limited exposure is required to apply the blade plate. (B) The blade plate allows for stable fixation even in the presence of metaphyseal comminution. (Courtesy of David Ring, M.D.)

5. Begin immediate passive and active-assisted range of motion in most patients following ORIF with a blade plate.

VI REHABILITATION

A Radiological Follow-Up

An initial postoperative radiographic evaluation including an AP and axillary view is required. The radiographs, including the same views, are repeated 2 weeks after surgery. In the absence of complications, final radiographs at 6 weeks postoperatively are sufficient and usually demonstrate a healed fracture.

B Rehabilitation

Postoperative rehabilitation depends on the technique used for stabilization and the quality of fixation. If percutaneous pinning has been used after open reduction, the postoperative management does not differ from closed reduction and percutaneous pinning.

Blade plate fixation has the advantage of providing excellent fixation even in elderly patients with poor bone quality. This allows for immediate passive and active-assisted range of motion. If the fracture is healing on the x-ray performed

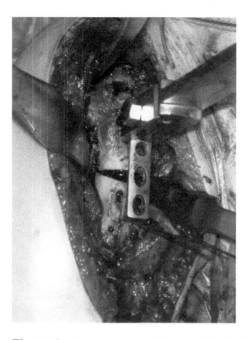

Figure 9   After proper positioning of the blade in the humeral head, the proximal fragment can be manipulated with the plate holder without additional soft tissue dissection (here in the case of an osteotomy).

2 weeks after surgery, more aggressive stretching and active range of motion can be started from the third week postoperatively.

REFERENCES

1. Alnot JY. Paralytic shoulder secondary to post-traumatic peripheral nerve lesions in the adult. Acta Orthop Belg 1999; 65:10–22.
2. Bigliani LU. Treatment of two- and three-part fractures of the proximal humerus. Instr Course Lect 1989; 38:231–244.
3. Bonnard C, Anastakis DJ, van Melle G, Narakas AO. Isolated and combined lesions of the axillary nerve. A review of 146 cases. J Bone Joint Surg Br 1999; 81:212–217.
4. Bosworth DM. Blade plate fixation. JAMA 1949; 141:1111.
5. Chun J-M, Groh GI, Rockwood CA. Two-part fractures of the proximal humerus. J Shoulder Elbow Surg 1994; 5:273–287.
6. Clifford PC. Fractures of the neck of the humerus: a review of the late results. Injury 1980; 12:91–95.
7. Coudane H, Fays J, Quiévreux P, et al. Fractures de l'extrémité supérieure de l'humérus. Conséquence sur la vascularisation céphalique. Cahiers d'enseignement de la SOFCOT 1996; 56:38–41.
8. Gerber C, Warner J, Alternatives to hemiarthroplasty for complex proximal- humeral fractures. In: Warner JJ, Iannotti JP, Gerber C, eds. Complex and Revision Problems in Shoulder Surgery. Philadelphia: Lippincott-Raven, 1997:215–243.
9. Hintermann B, Trouillier HH, Schafer D. Rigid internal fixation of fractures of the proximal humerus in older patients. J Bone Joint Surg Br 2000; 82:1107–1112.

10. Jaberg H, Warner JJ, Jakob RP. Percutaneous stabilization of unstable fractures of the humerus. J Bone Joint Surg Am 1992; 74:508–515.

11. Jakob R, Ganz R. Proximale Humerusfrakturen. Helv Chir Acta 1981; 48:595–610.

12. Jakob RP, Miniaci A, Anson PS, et al. Four-part valgus impacted fractures of the proximal humerus. J Bone Joint Surg Br 1991; 73:295–298.

13. Jupiter JB, Mullaji AB. Blade plate fixation of proximal humeral non-unions. Injury 1994; 25:301–303.

14. Kristiansen B, Kofoed H. External fixation of displaced fractures of the proximal humerus. Technique and preliminary results. J Bone Joint Surg Br 1987; 69:643–646.

15. Mouradian WH. Displaced proximal humeral fractures. Seven years' experience with a modified Zickel supracondylar device. Clin Orthop 1986; 212:209–218.

16. Neer CS. Shoulder Reconstruction. Philadelphia: WB Saunders, 1990.

17. Sehr JR, Szabo RM. Semitubular blade plate for fixation in the proximal humerus. J Orthop Trauma 1988; 4:327–332.

18. Sturzenegger M, Fornaro E, Jakob RP. Results of surgical treatment of multifragmented fractures of the humeral head. Arch Orthop Trauma Surg 1982; 100:249–259.

19. Wheeler DL, Colville MR. Biomechanical comparison of intramedullary and percutaneous pin fixation for proximal humeral fracture fixation. J Orthop Trauma 1997; 11:363–367.

20. Zuckerman JD, Flugstad DL, Teitz CC, King HA. Axillary artery injury as a complication of proximal humeral fractures. Clin Orthop 1984; 189:234–237.

5

Open Reduction and Internal Fixation of Three-Part Proximal Humerus Fractures

LEESA M. GALATZ and KEN YAMAGUCHI

Washington University School of Medicine and Barnes-Jewish Hospital, St. Louis, Missouri, U.S.A.

I INTRODUCTION

Open reduction and internal fixation (ORIF) is the standard initial method of treatment for most displaced, unstable three-part proximal humerus fractures. Multiple types of fixation have been described, specifically intramedullary rods, intramedullary rods with cerclage wire or suture, blade plate, T-plate, and, finally, tension band fixation (1–9). Successful results have been described using all these methods, but certain methods have emerged as superior in terms of stability and complication rates.

Factors considered in clinical decision making include patient age, activity level, and bone quality. These factors can directly influence the decision as to operative versus nonoperative treatment and whether or not open reduction and internal fixation is appropriate. Inability to obtain secure fixation in osteoporotic bone may preclude any of these methods of open reduction and internal fixation. In these cases, a hemiarthroplasty may be more appropriate. Stable fixation is critical for a successful outcome after ORIF of any proximal humerus fracture.

This chapter will review the many methods described for the fixation of three-part proximal humerus fractures. Concentration will be placed on the authors' preferred method as well as many pearls and pitfalls associated with the procedure. Most three-part proximal humerus fractures are amenable to operative fixation, and with careful attention to detail and good operative technique, restoration of the normal anatomy of the proximal humerus is possible.

II PREOPERATIVE PLANNING

A Patient Evaluation

Proximal humerus fractures usually occur in the elderly population (10). Risk factors identified in this population include poor bone quality, impaired vision and balance, medical comorbidities, and decreased muscle tone and strength (11). Fractures often result from a fall onto an outstretched hand and also occur after a direct blow to the lateral aspect of the shoulder, either from the floor or an object onto which they have fallen (12). Proximal humerus fractures in younger people with good bone stock usually result from high-energy injuries. The mechanism is often a motorized vehicle accident or a fall from a height. Seizures and electrocution are potential indirect mechanisms of proximal humerus fractures, but these are rare. Mechanism of injury influences choice of treatment method (8). In a young person with good bone quality, every attempt should be made at open reduction and internal fixation in order to restore anatomy and preserve native bone (6). In an older person, medical comorbidities may preclude surgery (6). Poor bone quality may make stable fracture fixation difficult or impossible.

B Physical Examination

Every patient with a proximal humerus fracture needs a thorough physical examination of the affected extremity. Emphasis is placed on neurological evaluation. The incidence of neurological injury after proximal humerus fractures is relatively high, especially in older patients with significant hematoma formation. Neurological injury occurs in 21–45% of proximal humerus fractures in these studies. The most common nerves affected are the axillary, musculocutaneous, suprascapular, and radial nerves (13). Most patients recover completely from the initial neurological deficit; however, a small percentage have persistent motor loss.

Vascular examination is equally important, as arterial injury constitutes a surgical emergency. Twenty-seven percent of patients with major arterial injuries about the shoulder can still have palpable pulses because of extensive collateral circulation between the shoulder and arm (14). The patient should be examined for any signs of ischemia distally, which when found should prompt a more thorough evaluation for vascular injury with arteriography.

Extensive ecchymoses can develop around the arm and elbow, and this can be associated with significant edema. Fracture blisters can develop as a result. Elderly patients are at increased risk for skin compromise due to fragile skin. When significant edema develops, it is useful to place the arm in a lymphedema stocking and compression glove to decrease swelling and protect the skin. The wrist and elbow should be carefully evaluated for any signs of concurrent injury.

C Radiographic Evaluation

Successful management depends on an accurate diagnosis made by radiographic examination. The three-part proximal humerus fracture generally involves the surgical neck of the humerus and the greater tuberosity. Rarely, the lesser tuberosity is involved. A standard x-ray series includes an anteroposterior view of the shoulder, a scapular anteroposterior view of the shoulder, an axillary view, and a scapular Y. The scapular AP and the axillary view are the most useful. An axillary view is particularly important because often the greater tuberosity fragment is displaced posteriorly and this is not always appreciated on the anteroposterior view. A standard axillary or Velpeau x-ray is also critical in ensuring the fracture is not associated with a dislocation.

Operative versus nonoperative treatment depends on the displacement of the fracture fragments. Neer (15,16) established the most commonly utilized parameters to describe displacement of proximal humerus fractures—1 cm of displacement and 45° of angulation. However, no study has directly correlated outcome after proximal humerus fracture with displacement. The most critical displacement is of the greater tuberosity relative to the humeral head. Superior displacement of the tuberosity fragment is not well tolerated.

Efficient biomechanical function of the rotator cuff is based on an anatomical relationship between the head and the tuberosity, such that adequate soft tissue tension of the cuff is maintained. Superior displacement of the greater tuberosity can result in subacromial impingement with overhead elevation. While 1 cm is the criteria for displacement, less displacement can be problematic. Operative treatment is considered at 5 mm (17), but definitive criteria have not been established. Because of the large range of motion of the shoulder in multiple planes, displacement at the surgical neck is better tolerated.

Extensive comminution at the metaphysis of the humerus can make a three-part proximal humerus fracture particularly unstable and presents a significant challenge when it involves a large portion of the proximal shaft of the humerus. As a result, it is difficult to obtain a stable construct when the proximal humeral shaft is reduced to the head. Stable reduction may require impaction of the shaft into the head, which will result in some shortening. If too much shortening is required, it may be necessary to augment with bone graft to obtain stability and maintain length.

The necessity for a CT scan is debatable. If a quality set of standard radiographs can be obtained, then it is generally not necessary. With adequate radiographs, fracture lines can be visualized and displacement is predictable based on muscle attachments to the fractured fragments. For example, at the surgical neck fracture, the shaft is displaced anteriorly and medially because of the force from the attached pectoralis major muscle. The greater tuberosity fragment is displaced posteriorly and medially by the rotator cuff. The head fragment is rotated internally by the subscapularis, which inserts on to the intact lesser tuberosity. However, if there is any question about the anatomy of the fracture or if there is a suspected head split component, then a CT scan may add useful information.

III OPERATIVE APPROACH

Multiple methods using several different types of hardware have been described for the operative fixation of three-part proximal humerus fractures. The use of intramedullary rods alone in three-part proximal humerus fractures is generally not recommended, as this does not give good fixation of the displaced greater tuberosity fragment or of the surgical neck fracture. Alternatively, intramedullary rods can be used in combination with cerclage wire or suture (2). Modified Enders rods have been used for this purpose as well. These rods are modified so that they have a small hole at the proximal end to facilitate passage of the figure of 8 suture allowing incorporation of the rod into the overall fixation. The rods are passed from proximal to distal down the shaft of the humerus through the unaffected tuberosity. The proximal tips of the nails are buried beneath the level of the tuberosity. The sutures are then passed through the tendon superiorly and then through holes in the proximal aspect of the humeral shaft. They are crossed and tied in figure-8 fashion. The biomechanical strength of this construct has been evaluated in cadaveric studies of surgical neck fractures (18). Mechanical irritation of the rotator cuff and subacromial impingement is one problem identified with the use of this method, often requiring later hardware removal.

Tension band fixation was described by Hawkins et al. (3). In this method the sutures are passed incorporating the rotator cuff tendon at the bone tendon junction at both the greater and lesser tuberosities with the use of a culposcopy needle. The sutures are crossed in figure-8 fashion and passed through drill holes in the proximal humeral shaft.

Standard T-plate fixation of the proximal humerus is another option, but it is often criticized because of high failure rates (4). Failure is largely due to the extensive soft tissue stripping necessary to apply the plate, inadequate screw purchase, and subacromial impingement by the plate. The potential for hardware impingement increases when the plate is placed superiorly along the lateral aspect of the humerus so that with arm elevation, the hardware becomes subacromial in position. Furthermore, loss of fixation of the humeral head that results in further varus displacement of the proximal fragment leads to increased prominence of the plate. Esser (9) reported good results, however, using a modified cloverleaf plate. He used smaller 4.0 mm cancellous screws instead of the larger 6.5 mm screws and attributed successful results to limited exposure and a more careful soft tissue dissection in order to preserve vascularity to the humeral head. The patient population also had good bone stock, another factor likely contributing to the successful results.

The authors utilize a method combining the techniques of percutaneous pinning (19) and cerclage suture (3). This method is appropriate for fractures in patients with adequate bone stock and minimal to no comminution of the metaphysis. Two or three pins are placed in retrograde fashion from the humeral shaft into the humeral head. Tension band sutures are passed through the lesser tuberosity and the greater tuberosity at the bone-tendon junction before crossing in figure-8 fashion. (Fig. 1) They can either be passed through drill holes in the humeral shaft or in some cases, tied around the percutaneous pins at the shaft. The greatest risk of this procedure is loss of fixation of the pins in the humeral head.

IV AUTHORS' PREFERRED METHOD

A Surgical Approach

The deltopectoral or extended deltopectoral approach is used for the treatment of three-part proximal humerus fractures. The incision is made from the tip of the coracoid, along the deltopectoral interval and at the most distal aspect angulates slightly laterally toward the deltoid insertion on the humerus. Identification of the deltopectoral interval is critical as failure to do so risks denervation of the anterior portion of the deltoid. The cephalic vein is retracted laterally with the deltoid. A deep self-retaining retractor is then placed in the deltopectoral interval. The plane underneath the deltoid is developed throughout the entire subacromial space and

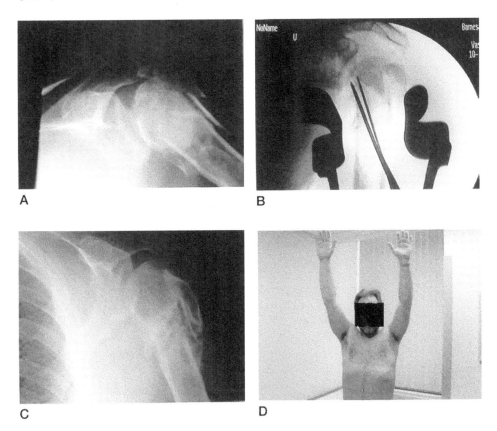

Figure 1   (A) A displaced three-part proximal humerus fracture in a 47-year-old male following a parachuting accident. (B) An intraoperative flouroscan of the same fracture after fixation with pins and tension band sutures. (C) An anteroposterior radiograph one year after surgery demonstrating the healed fracture. (D) One year after surgery, the patient could attain full overhead elevation.

posteriorly and laterally around the humerus. A free subdeltoid and subacromial space is critical for adequate visualization and mobilization of fragments. Care should be taken to protect the axillary nerve on the undersurface of the deltoid.

The lateral edge of the conjoined tendon is then identified, freed from hematoma and scar tissue, and incorporated in the self-retaining retractor. The retractor should not place excessive traction on the conjoined tendon in order to avoid traction on the musculocutaneous nerve or inadvertently injure the axillary nerve. At this point, adequate visualization of the proximal humerus is usually obtained. If necessary, however, additional exposure can be obtained by releasing the upper half of the pectoralis major insertion from the humerus just lateral to the bicipital groove. In some isolated, difficult cases where there is significant comminution of the upper portion of the humeral shaft, additional distal exposure can be obtained by raising a small amount of the anterior deltoid insertion from the humeral shaft. However, this is rarely necessary for routine three-part proximal humerus fractures.

B Surgical Technique

The first goal after exposure is to obtain control of the greater tuberosity fragment. Again, it is essential to have a complete release throughout the subacromial space and posteriorly around the humeral head and neck so that visualization and mobilization of the fragment is possible. A tagging suture is placed through the supraspinatus at the bone-tendon junction. This is used to assist with mobilization and positioning at the time of fixation. Care should be taken not to place this suture through the bone of the greater tuberosity itself. The tendon is much stronger, and there is a risk of fracture of the greater tuberosity fragment if a traction suture is passed through the bone. The greater tuberosity fragment is usually displaced posteriorly (Fig. 2A) and should be mobilized anteriorly in order to place it in an anatomical position.

Attention is then turned to the surgical neck fracture. The humeral shaft is reduced in anatomical position to the head fragment. It is often helpful to utilize fluoroscopy in the operating room at this point. The biceps tendon is a useful landmark, and it may be helpful to expose a portion of it as it traverses superiorly in order to ensure that the head is appropriately aligned with the shaft. The biceps tendon courses more anteriorly as it proceeds distally along the shaft. This should be taken into consideration when evaluating correct rotational alignment. The normal angle of inclination between the anatomical neck and humeral shaft is approximately 35–40°. The humeral head is retroverted 20–30°. These measurements are important during reduction, as malunion is associated with inferior results.

When there is mild comminution of the metaphysis, the shaft should be impacted into the head fragment in order to obtain some stability. Some shortening will occur as a result; however, it is virtually impossible to balance a head fragment on the tip of pins without good contact between the head fragment and the shaft. The pins are then placed from the shaft into the humeral head (Fig. 2B). If severe comminution of the metaphysis precludes a stable reduction or results in excessive shortening, the authors recommend plate fixation as an alternative (see below).

The location of pin placement is critical (7,19). The pins should enter the humerus above the deltoid insertion. Pins are placed in two different directions, and the starting point for the pins on the humeral shaft should not be too close. One pin is placed from the lateral aspect of the shaft up into the head, and the second pin is placed in a more anterior-posterior direction. Pin placement and stability should be checked under fluoroscopy. The pins can usually be placed through the skin incision; however, occasionally a small accessory skin incision may be necessary for proper pin orientation and alignment.

Size 2.7 or 2.5 mm terminally threaded pins are used in this procedure. The threaded tip enhances fixation in the humeral head. Fully threaded pins are avoided because they wind soft tissue during implantation, risking injury to the deltoid muscle and the axillary nerve. Axillary nerve injury can be avoided with placement in an open procedure where the pins can be visualized at their entrance point into the humerus through the incision. A large drill guide can be used as a canula for the pin if there is any concern about where it traverses the deltoid.

Fixation of the greater tuberosity fragment is obtained using heavy suture (Fig. 2C) The authors' prefer no. 1 cottony Dacron (Deknatel, Fall River, MA) or no. 5 Ethibond (Ethicon, Somerville, NJ). The greater tuberosity is mobilized by releasing

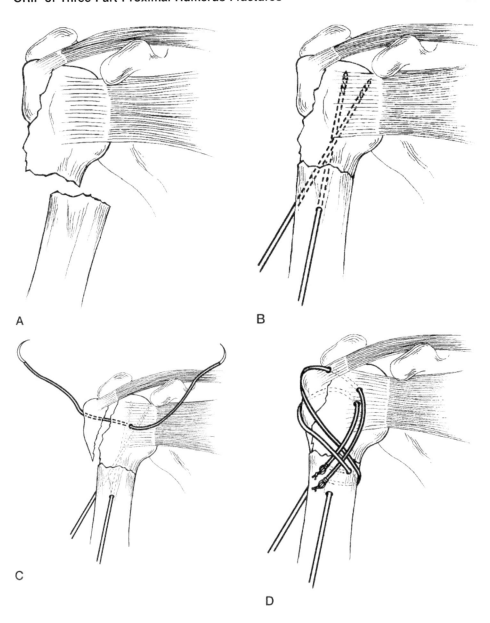

Figure 2 (A) A diagram representative of a three-part proximal humerus fracture demonstrating anterior and medial displacement of the shaft secondary to the force of the attached pectoralis major muscle, superior and posterior displacement of the greater tuberosity fragment with its attached rotator cuff, and the remainder of the humeral head fragment with the subscapularis attached to the lesser tuberosity. (B) After the humeral head is reduced to the shaft, two terminally threaded 2.7 mm pins are placed in retrograde fashion stabilizing the reduction. (C) Fixation of the greater tuberosity is obtained with heavy suture, placing the suture at the bone-tendon junction of the greater and the lesser tuberosity before crossing in figure-8 fashion. (D) The sutures are crossed in figure-8 fashion and passed through drill holes in the humeral shaft, creating a tension band across the fracture site.

it from any early scar in the subacromial space. Opening the rotator interval is helpful for mobilizing and reducing the fragment. Two sutures are placed through the posterior rotator cuff at the bone-tendon junction. The other limbs are brought through the subscapularis bone-tendon junction. They are crossed in figure-8 fashion. The sutures are passed through drill holes in the humeral shaft and then tied, securing the greater tuberosity to the shaft and creating a tension band across the fracture site (Fig. 2D). The pins are cut just below the level of the skin to avoid irritation and possible skin tract infections. Reduction should be evaluated by an anteroposterior x-ray in the operating room before completion of the procedure.

The biceps tendon is a potential source of pain after tension band fixation of proximal humerus fractures because it directly underlies the sutures that are secured tightly over the intertubercular groove. Concern over this issue is debatable. Some prefer to leave the biceps in place, allowing it to autotenodese in the groove. It is the authors' preference to perform a tenotomy as proximally as possible and tenodese the biceps in the groove. The wound is then irrigated and closed over suction drainage.

Some fractures may not be amenable to this method of fixation in spite of good bone stock because of extensive comminution at the metaphysis (Fig. 3A). A blade or modified clover leaf plate may be a better option in these patients. A plate offers stability across the comminuted fracture site in situations where good screw purchase can be obtained in the humeral head. Minimal soft tissue dissection in the area of the ascending branch of the anterior humeral circumflex artery should be performed in order to preserve vascularity to the humeral head. This is usually easy to avoid because the artery courses along the lateral aspect of the intertubercular groove, which usually stays with the lesser tuberosity and head fragment.

Satisfactory results have been reported with either a blade (5) or a cloverleaf plate (9). The modified cloverleaf plate offers the advantage of allowing several screws to obtain fixation in the head. The superior aspect of the plate is positioned well inferior to the top of the greater tuberosity in order to avoid mechanical impingement in the subacromial space with overhead elevation. We prefer the use of 4.0 mm screws as described by Esser (9). On some occasions, autologous bone

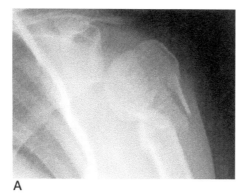 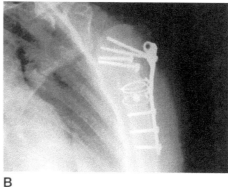

A   B

Figure 3   (A) A three-part proximal humerus fracture with extensive comminution of the metaphysis. (B) Fixation of this fracture with a modified cloverleaf plate utilizing an iliac crest bone graft strut inserted into the humeral shaft and impacted into the head.

grafting with iliac crest is helpful in providing stability across a comminuted proximal shaft (Fig. 3B). The graft is placed in the shaft and impacted into the head fragment, but this is rarely necessary in acute fractures. If stable ORIF of the three-part proximal humerus cannot be obtained, a hemiarthroplasty should be considered.

V PEARLS AND PITFALLS

A Pearls

Several important points deserve emphasis with regard to this technique. The first relates to pin placement. The pins should be placed in different directions at least 1 cm from each other at the entry point. One pin enters laterally and is directed medially and posteriorly into the humeral head. The other begins more anteriorly on the shaft and courses posteriorly and medially. Close, parallel pins act as a single point of fixation allowing rotation around the two pins. Pins further from each other at the entry point and in two different directions create a stronger construct. The normal retroversion of the humeral head should be taken into consideration during pin placement to keep from cutting out of the head.

At least one suture for fixation of the greater tuberosity should be placed at the bone-tendon junction and not through the bone. This is the strongest area in the rotator cuff tendon–greater tuberosity construct. Placement of sutures through the greater tuberosity itself increases the risk of fracturing the fragment. This bone is often quite soft, especially in elderly individuals.

Suture attachment to the humeral shaft itself can be difficult. We generally prefer attachment through drill holes in the humerus, but if the patient has good bone stock and the surgeon is confident in pin fixation, the sutures can be tied around the pins. Another option, if suture placement to the shaft is difficult, is to place a screw across the humerus, leaving the head of the screw as a post around which the sutures are tied.

Injury to the axillary nerve on the undersurface of the deltoid is avoided by careful placement of the pins. Often through this open approach they can be placed under direct visualization. A large drill guide placed along the bone is also used for protection.

B Pitfalls

A major pitfall is placing the pins too close to one another and in the same direction. This allows rotation at the fracture site around the pins. This technique should not be used in osteoporotic patients with insufficient bone stock in the humeral head. The bone of the tuberosity is soft and suture cut-out likely if tension band sutures are not placed at the bone tendon junction. Malunion of the tuberosity leads to poorer outcome and usually results from inadequate mobilization and fixation. The level of the tuberosity should be 5–8 mm below the level of the humeral head. Superior displacement will result in subacromial impingement with arm elevation.

Stability is assessed by direct visualization at the completion of the procedure. Any suggestion of instability at the fracture site with gentle range of motion is unacceptable, and another procedure such as plate fixation or hemiarthroplasty should be considered. If there is significant bone loss or comminution associated with the fracture, autologous bone grafting with a section of tricortical iliac crest may be necessary to obtain stability between the head and the shaft. This is preferable to excessive shortening.

VI POSTOPERATIVE REHABILITATION

Postoperatively, the patient is placed in a sling. X-rays are taken every 7–10 days for the first 3 weeks. New sets of radiographs are obtained at 6 weeks, 3 months, 6 months, and 1 year unless circumstances dictate otherwise. The pins should be left for a minimum of 3 weeks and are removed ideally after 6 weeks. They often cause discomfort to the patient, and we advise them of this preoperatively. The pins are usually removed quite easily during a sterile office procedure. If there is any concern about the ability to do this in the office or because of patient apprehension, removal can be performed in the operating room.

Physical therapy is initiated immediately postoperatively. Early initiation of rehabilitation is associated with improved recovery during the first 3 months after surgery (20). Gentle pendulum exercises begin on postoperative day 1. Passive range-of-motion exercises are initiated during the first week as well. Specifically, this consists of passive supine forward flexion, passive external rotation with the arm at the side, and pendulum exercises. The patient is instructed to place a pillow under the elbow to keep the shoulder from going into extension when in a supine position, maintaining the arm at the midplane of the body. At 6 weeks or when there are signs of healing, the patient progresses to active range of motion and light strengthening shortly thereafter. If there is a question about consolidation of the fracture at the 6-week point, then active range of motion is delayed. The rehabilitation program progresses to advanced stretching and strengthening with resistive weights and bands at 12 weeks. Patients can continue to improve for 12–18 months, so exercise protocols should extend throughout this period.

VII RESULTS

Overall, results reported in the literature following ORIF are satisfactory in the majority of patients. However, studies are somewhat difficult to interpret and compare to each other because the series are generally small and not randomized. It is difficult to control for severity of injury, bone quality, treatment method, and surgeon skill and selection bias. Although some success with nonoperative treatment has been reported for displaced three-part fractures, Neer (15) reported no successful results in 20 three-part fractures treated with closed reduction. On the other hand, 19 of 31 patients treated operatively by Neer (16) had excellent or satisfactory results. He attributed the poor results to inadequate fixation. Currently, ORIF is the treatment of choice for displaced three-part fractures uncomplicated by age, bone quality, and patient health factors.

Successful results are reported for many different types of fixation. Cuomo et al. (2) demonstrated 100% satisfactory results after ORIF in eight patients with an average forward elevation to 150 degrees using Ender nails and tension band. Paavolainen et al. (4) reported 74% satisfactory results in 14 three-part fractures treated operatively with screws alone or with plate and screw fixation. Hawkins et al. (3) reported 87% satisfactory results using tension band wire technique in 15 patients. Thirteen percent developed osteonecrosis of the humeral head. Forward elevation averaged 126° in this older population (average age 60). Hintermann et al. (5) used blade plate fixation in 34 three-part fractures and 8 four-part fractures in a group of patients with an average age of 72 years. All the fractures healed. Avascular necrosis occurred in two. There were 30 good or excellent results.

Percutaneous pinning (7,19,21) and indirect reduction (22) methods have gained increased attention of late because of the potential to minimize soft tissue disruption and subsequent osteonecrosis. Hessman et al. (22) retrospectively reviewed a series of 98 patients after indirect reduction and plate fixation of unstable two-, three-, and four-part fractures with good to excellent results in 76%. Resch (7) originally described percutaneous pinning of proximal humerus fractures. Jaberg (19) recommends two pins through the greater tuberosity fragment engaging the medial cortex in addition to the retrograde pins from the shaft into the head.

T-plate fixation has been criticized (4) for high complication rates such as osteonecrosis, mechanical impingement from superior placement of the plate, loss of fixation, and malunion. However, Esser (9) treated 26 patients, 16 with three-part fractures, with a modified cloverleaf plate. The plate was malleable and conformed better to the proximal humerus than a rigid T-plate. Four mm screws were used in place of the larger 6.5 mm screws. There was less impingement with this plate and a very low failure rate. Taken together, these studies support ORIF as the initial treatment for three-part fractures of the proximal humerus in the majority of cases.

VIII CONCLUSION

Surgical management of three-part proximal humerus fractures is difficult and requires familiarity with more than one method of fixation. Poor bone quality, degree of comminution, and fracture displacement are factors that contribute to the complexity and difficulty of treating these fractures. Choice of fixation method is influenced by these factors. The pinning and tension band suture technique described here offers the advantage of combining the stability of the tension band technique with the added rigidity of pinning without requiring extensive dissection associated with use of a plate. There is no potential for mechanical impingement or irritation of the rotator cuff, often associated with other types of hardware.

Successful ORIF of three-part proximal humerus fractures requires anatomical reduction with careful soft tissue dissection and preservation of remaining humeral head vascularity, rigid fixation, and carefully timed, supervised rehabilitation. In general, vascularity is preserved with these fractures and rates of avascular necrosis are low. Results after operative fixation of fractures are satisfactory in a high percentage of patients in reported series, with anatomical reduction associated with a better outcome. Results are also improved when stable fixation allows earlier passive motion exercises. Rehabilitation requires physician supervision and patient cooperation.

REFERENCES

1. Cornell CN, Levine D, Pagnani MJ. Internal fixation of proximal humerus fractures using the screw-tension band technique. J Orthop Trauma 1994; 8:23–27.

2. Cuomo F, Flatow EL, Maday MG, et al. Open reduction and internal fixation of two- and three-part displaced surgical neck fractures of the proximal humerus. J Shoulder Elbow Surg 1992; 1:287–295.

3. Hawkins RJ, Bell RH, Gurr K. The three-part fracture of the proximal part of the humerus. J Bone Joint Surg 1986; 68A:1410–1414.

4. Paavolainen P. Operative treatment of severe proximal humeral fractures. Acta Orthop Scand 1983; 54:374–379.

5. Hintermann B, Trouillier H, Schafer D. Rigid internal fixation of fractures of the proximal humerus in older patients. J Bone Joint Surg Br 2000; 82:1107–1112.

6. Naranja R, Iannotti J. Displaced three- and four-part proximal humerus fractures: evaluation and management. J Am Acad Orthop Surg 2000; 8:373–382.

7. Resch H, Beck E, Bayley I. Reconstruction of the valgus-impacted humeral head fracture. J Shoulder Elbow Surg 1995; 4:73–80.

8. Williams G, Wong K. Two-part and three-part fractures: open reduction and internal fixation versus closed reduction and percutaneous pinning. Orthop Clin North Am 2000; 31:1–21.

9. Esser RD. Treatment of three- and four-part fractures of the proximal humerus with a modified cloverleaf plate. J Orthop Trauma 1994; 8:15–22.

10. Kannus P, Palvanen M, Niemi S, Parkkari J. Osteoporotic fractures of the proximal humerus in elderly Finnish persons: sharp increase in 1970–1998 and alarming projections for the new millennium. Acta Orthop Scand 2000; 71:465–470.

11. Nordqvist A, Petersson C. Incidence and causes of shoulder girdle injuries in an urban population. J Shoulder Elbow Surg 1995; 4:107–112.

12. Palvanen M, Kannus P, Parkkari J, Pitkajarvi T. The injury mechanisms of osteoporotic upper extremity fractures among older adults: a controlled study of 287 consecutive patients and their 108 controls. Osteoporos Int 2000; 11:822–831.

13. de Laat E, Visser C, Coene L, al e. Nerve lesions in primary shoulder dislocations and humeral neck fractures: a prospective clinical and EMG study. J Bone Joint Surg 1994; 76B:381–383.

14. Cuomo F. Proximal humerus fractures in elderly, American Academy of Orthopaedic Surgeons Annual Meeting, Instructional Course Lecture #247, San Francisco, CA, February 14, 1997.

15. Neer CSII. Displaced proximal humerus fractures. Part I. Classification and evaluation. J Bone Joint Surg 1970; 52A:1077–1089.

16. Neer CSII. Displaced proximal humeral fractures. Treatment of three-part and four-part displacement. J Bone Joint Surg 1970; 52:1090–1103.

17. McLaughlin HL. Posterior dislocation of the shoulder. J Bone Joint Surg 1952; 34A:584–590.

18. Williams GJ, Copley L, Iannotti J, Lesser S. The influence of figure-of-eight wiring for surgical neck fractures of the proximal humerus: a biomechanical study. J Shoulder Elbow Surg 1997; 6:423–428.

19. Jaberg H, Warner JJP, Jakob RP. Percutaneous stablization of unstable fractures of the humerus. J Bone Joint Surg 1992; 74-A:508–515.

20. Kristiansen B, Angermann P, Larsen TK. Functional results following fractures of the proximal humerus. Arch Orthop Trauma Surg 1989; 108:339–341.

21. Soete P, Clayson P, Costenoble V. Transitory percutaneous pinning in fractures of the proximal humerus. J Shoulder Elbow Surg 1999; 8:569–573.

22. Hessman M, Baumgaertel F, Gehling H. Plate fixation of proximal humeral fractures with indirect reduction: surgical technique and results utilizing three shoulder scores. Injury 1999; 30:453–462.

6

Open Reduction and Internal Fixation of Four-Part Proximal Humerus Fractures

ANDREAS M. SAUERBREY

Orthopedics of Steamboat Springs, Steamboat Springs, Colorado, U.S.A.

GERALD R. WILLIAMS, JR.

University of Pennsylvania School of Medicine, Philadelphia, Pennsylvania, U.S.A.

I OPERATIVE INDICATIONS

Four-part fractures typically occur in elderly patients with poor bone quality and are often not amenable to osteosynthesis. Avascular necrosis with subsequent collapse is common (1,2). Moreover, the results of hemiarthroplasty in this patient population are better than the results of operative fracture stabilization (1,3). Therefore, the optimal treatment for most four-part proximal humerus fractures is prosthetic replacement.

Classical four-part fractures may also occur in young patients as the result of high-energy trauma. These patients often have very active lifestyles that are not compatible with prosthetic management. Therefore, open reduction and internal fixation of proximal humerus fractures with four-part displacement is considered in patients under the age of 40. However, patient selection is critical to success. One must be able to obtain stable enough fixation to allow passive mobilization within the first postoperative week, and the patient must be reliable enough to cooperate with postoperative rehabilitation.

Valgus-impacted four-part fractures represent a special type of four-part fracture. They often are not comminuted and have a much lower incidence of avascular necrosis than classical four-part fractures because of arterial vessels that enter the head through the intact inferomedial periosteum (4). Consequently, operative stabilization is the preferred treatment of valgus-impacted four-part fractures, except in patients whose bone quality is too poor to obtain stable fixation.

Surgical management of acute valgus-impacted four-part fractures commonly involves closed or percutaneous reduction and percutaneous stabilization with pins and/or screws. This technique is predicated on the ability of the surgeon to obtain adequate reduction and fixation using closed or percutaneous means (see Chap. 2). The following chapter discusses open reduction and internal fixation of acute valgus-impacted four-part fractures that are not amenable to closed or percutaneous methods, subacute (> 2 weeks) valgus-impacted four-part fractures, and classical four-part fractures in patients under the age of 40.

II PREOPERATIVE PLANNING

Preoperative planning begins with an accurate diagnosis of the fracture and all other associated injuries. As mentioned above, four-part fractures in patients under the age of 40 are often the result of high-energy trauma. Therefore, physical examination is directed toward identifying more serious injuries such as chest or rib injuries, intra-abdominal injuries, or intracranial injuries. In addition, a musculoskeletal survey should be performed to identify spine, pelvic, or other long bone fractures. Motor function should be verified in all five (axillary, musculocutaneous, radial, median, and ulnar) major peripheral nerve distributions of the injured upper extremity, as sensory examination around the shoulder is unreliable. A high index of suspicion must be maintained with regard to associated axillary arterial injury because of the extensive collateral circulation between the third part of the subclavian artery and the third part of the axillary artery (5).

The decision to proceed with open reduction and internal fixation of a four-part proximal humerus fracture is based not only on patient age and activity level but also on degree of comminution and integrity of the articular segment. If the humeral head is fractured into two or more pieces, anatomical reduction and stable fixation may not be possible. The importance of the trauma series of radiographs in accurately classifying the fracture cannot be overemphasized (see Chap. 1). If adequate assessment of the fracture cannot be obtained with plain radiographs, computed tomographic (CT) scanning is indicated. Three-dimensional reconstruction of the axial CT images is not mandatory but may aid in determining the displacement and orientation of the head fragment. In the vast majority of cases, however, the fracture can be adequately characterized and a treatment plan can be formulated on the basis of the trauma series alone. A CT scan should not be a substitute for poor radiographs.

Multiple fixation methods have been described for osteosynthesis of proximal humerus fractures. These methods include interfragmentary sutures or wires, tension band wires, pins, screws, plates, blade-plates, and intramedullary rods. None of these methods is ideal for all fractures. Therefore, the surgeon must be familiar with more than one method and plan to have the appropriate instruments and/or implants available in the operating room. From a practical standpoint, one should have heavy nonabsorbable suture material, wire (18 gauge or bigger), multiple sized kirschner wires, terminally threaded 2.5 mm pins (guidewires from the 6.5 mm cannulated screw set), Ender's rods, and a plate/blade-plate and screw fixation system. A small (4.0–4.5 mm) cannulated screw system may facilitate the fixation process but is not essential.

Impaction or actual partial loss of the metaphyseal cancelleous bone of the proximal humerus is common in four-part fractures, particularly those involving valgus impaction of the humeral head. Once the head and tuberosities have been returned to their anatomical positions, deficiency of the metaphyseal bone may exist. Although reconstitution of this defect is not required in all cases, preoperative planning must include the potential for use of cancelleous bone graft or other bone substitutes. A detailed discussion of the risks and benefits of cancelleous autograft, cancelleous allograft, and the multitude of bone substitutes available is beyond the scope of this chapter. However, the possible need for these materials and the potential ramifications of their use should be discussed with the patient and his or her family preoperatively. Moreover, arrangements should be made with the operating room to have cancelleous allograft bone chips or whatever other bone substitute has been decided upon available.

Fracture reduction is often difficult to visualize intraoperatively. The rotator cuff inserts extensively on the greater and lesser tuberosities and makes visualization of the head and other fracture fragments difficult. Although incision of the rotator interval may improve visualization of the joint and articular surface of the head fragment, intraoperative assessment of the reduction may still be difficult. Therefore, preoperative arrangements should be made for intraoperative use of a C-arm and image intensifier. If a C-arm is not available, intraoperative plain radiographs may be obtained.

Operative stabilization of any four-part proximal humerus fracture should never be undertaken without the ability to convert to a hemiarthroplasty intraoperatively. The surgeon may find that the degree of comminution and severity of the injury were underestimated preoperatively and that stable fixation is not possible. This possibility should have been discussed with the patient and his or her family preoperatively. Moreover, a shoulder arthroplasty instrument set and a complete set of implants should be available in the operating room.

III OPERATIVE APPROACHES

A Valgus-Impacted Four-Part Fractures

1 Acute Valgus-Impacted Fracture

As mentioned previously, the majority of acute valgus-impacted four-part fractures are amenable to closed or percutaneous reduction and percutaneous fixation. Although this technique is discussed in detail in Chapter two, certain aspects of the technique are emphasized here because they are also relevant to open reduction and internal fixation. The musculo-periosteal sleeve surrounding the tuberosities is intact. Therefore, when tension in the sleeve is reestablished by reducing the head, the tuberosities reduce easily. The head is maintained in its reduced position with retrograde 2.5 mm terminally threaded pins inserted through the anterolateral shaft into the head. The tuberosities are stabilized either with 2.5 mm terminally threaded pins or cannulated screws placed percutaneously (Fig. 1).

If the head cannot be reduced percutaneously, open reduction and internal fixation is indicated. Both deltopectoral and deltoid-splitting approaches have been described (6). The lateral, deltoid-splitting approach offers the advantage of better visualization of the greater tuberosity fracture line. However, this approach cannot be extended more than 4.5–5.0 cm distal to the lateral margin of the acromion

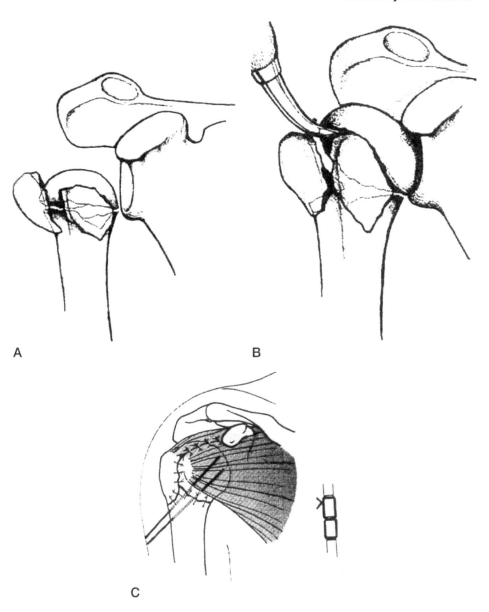

Figure 1 Valgus-impacted four-part fractures are characterized by valgus impaction of the head onto the shaft with separation of the tuberosities to allow head displacement (A). During open reduction, the head is elevated back into its normal position and the tuberosities reduce spontaneously (B). Retrograde pins from the shaft to the reduced head maintain the reduction (C). The tuberosities are stabilized with interfragmentary sutures that cross within the fractures to discourage overreduction (C, inset). (From Ref. 4.)

without damaging the axillary nerve. Therefore, it is not as versatile as the deltopectoral approach.

Once the fracture is exposed, two basic methods of reduction and stabilization have been described. One method involves extensive dissection of the fracture fragments, direct fracture reduction, and plate/screw fixation. The other method involves minimal surgical dissection, indirect reduction of the tuberosities by reducing the head with an elevator placed through the gap between the tuberosities, and minimal internal fixation using a combination of terminally threaded pins, screws, and interfragmentary sutures. Cancelleous bone grafting has been described with both methods (6–8).

2 Subacute (> 2 weeks) Valgus-Impacted Fractures

Valgus-impacted four-part fractures begin to heal quickly because of the stability imparted by the impaction and the type of bone through which they occur. Consequently, fractures that are more than 2 weeks old will be difficult to reduce percutaneously without applying significant force to the head fragment. Maintaining the inferomedial periosteal vessels is important in minimizing the risk of avascular necrosis. The reduction is probably more safely obtained through open means. The approaches, reduction, and fixation options are the same as in the acute situation. The use of cancelleous bone graft or bone substitute is more likely in the subacute setting because there is a greater tendency for the head to collapse into varus. This may be the result of scarring and early contracture of the musculo-periosteal sleeve.

B Classical Four-Part Fractures

Open reduction and internal fixation of standard four-part fractures is performed through a deltopectoral approach. Multiple methods of fixation have been described. These methods fall under three general categories: intramedullary, extramedullary—plate osteosynthesis, and extramedullary—minimal osteosynthesis.

Intramedullary devices may be rigid or flexible. Fixation of the proximal fracture fragments is typically obtained with screws that pass through the nail or wires passed in a tension band configuration. Mouradian used a modification of the Zickel nail—described for supracondylar femur fractures—to treat a variety of proximal humerus fractures, seven of which were four-part fractures (9). Darder et al. used intramedullary K-wires reinforced with a tension band wire in a series of 33 displaced four-part fractures. The K-wires were passed through the tuberosities and down the shaft, and the tension band was passed between the tuberosity K-wires to the shaft (10).

Plates have also been advocated in the treatment of true four-part fractures. Techniques have been described for T-plates (11,12), cloverleaf plates (13,14), and blade-plates (15). The two major disadvantages of plate fixation are the soft-tissue dissection required to place the plate and impingement of the upper margin of the plate against the acromion. Esser (13) reported the use of a modified cloverleaf plate in the treatment of 10 four-part fractures. The plate was modified by removing the superior and anterior portions of the cloverleaf. These modifications may help to avoid subacromial impingement and injury to the ascending branch of the anterior humeral circumflex artery, the terminal branch of which (arcuate artery) supplies the major portion of the humeral head blood supply. The advantages of the cloverleaf plate are the ability to place multiple screws into the head fragment and the ability to contour the plate to fit the anatomical configuration of the proximal-lateral humerus. Early screw pullout from the humeral head with loss of reduction has been reported following open reduction and internal fixation with plates and screws (12).

However, appropriate patient selection to avoid patients with poor bone quality may decrease this complication.

Extramedullary stabilization with minimal internal fixation offers the potential advantage of less soft tissue dissection. This theoretically could result in a lower incidence of avascular necrosis. The disadvantage, however, is that fixation may be suboptimal and prevent early motion. These types of extramedullary fixation include pins, screws, tension band or figure-8 wires, and combinations of these methods (16).

IV MY PERSONAL APPROACH

The goal of operative stabilization of any four-part fracture is an anatomical reduction. There is no one correct method to achieve this. Moreover, as one's experience with operative treatment of proximal humerus fractures in general increases, preferred operative techniques may mature or change. This section is meant to be a guide to one person's method of four-part fracture management at one point in time. As the reader encounters patients in his or her own practice with four-part fractures requiring operative stabilization, hopefully these thoughts will provide a backdrop of sound surgical principles that lead to anatomical reduction and stable fixation, even if the exact techniques are not the same.

All four-part fractures are stabilized through an anterior deltopectoral approach. Therefore, anesthesia, patient set-up, and superficial surgical approach are the same for all fracture types. Although the choice of anesthetic is made by the patient after a discussion with the anesthesiologist, combined general anesthesia and interscalene block allows for maximum intraoperative control and postoperative pain management.

After adequate anesthesia has been obtained, the operating table is placed in the semi-recumbent position with the back of the table elevated 30–45°. The entire shoulder girdle must be unsupported off the edge of the operating table to ensure that adequate radiographs can be obtained and that the arm can be adducted and extended enough to allow placement of a humeral prosthesis if necessary. This can be accomplished by lateralizing the entire patient on a standard operating table so that the shoulder and arm extend over the edge. Alternatively, special operating tables exist that have panels on either side that can be removed to expose the ipsilateral shoulder girdle. Whichever table is used, a padded retaining post should be attached to the table and rest against the thorax to prevent inadvertent pulling of the patient off the table (Fig. 2A).

The C-arm and image intensifier are brought into the operating room and positioned appropriately. The C-arm should be positioned at the head of the table, parallel to the lateral edge of the table. This will require that the anesthesiologist and his or her equipment be moved over near the opposite extremity (Fig. 2B). The ability to obtain an anterior-posterior and axillary view should be verified before the surgical field is prepared and draped (Fig. 3).

A skin incision is made parallel to the deltopectoral interval. The length of the incision depends upon the proposed fixation plan. If minimal internal fixation methods are planned, the incision may extend 6–8 cm from slightly superior and medial to the tip of the coracoid toward the deltoid tuberosity. If plate fixation is contemplated, a more extensile incision is required and the incision described above is carried distally, all the way to the deltoid tuberosity (Fig. 4). The cephalic vein is

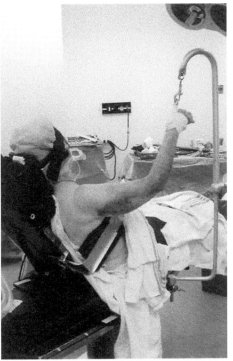
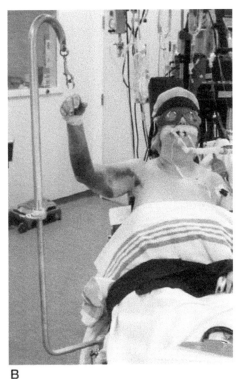

A   B

Figure 2 The patient is placed in the beach chair position with the head elevated 30–40°. The arm should extend over the edge of the table so that the superior, posterior, and anterior aspects of the shoulder can be accessed. This also allows extension, adduction, and external rotation should access to the humeral canal be required to place a humeral prosthesis. A lateral post prevents inadvertent pulling of the patient off the table (A). The anesthesia equipment is displaced to the opposite side to allow the surgeon or the C-arm to come in from the superior aspect of the shoulder (B).

separated from the pectoralis major and retracted laterally with the deltoid. In most cases, both the deltoid origin and insertion can be preserved. If a plate or blade-plate is utilized, a small portion of the most anterior fibers of the deltoid insertion may need to be released. The clavipectoral fascia is incised lateral to the conjoined tendon of the coracobrachialis and short head of the biceps; the coracoacromial ligament is preserved. The biceps tendon is identified, deep to the pectoralis major tendon, as a guide to the bicipital groove and tuberosity fragments. At this point the surgical approach changes, based upon the fracture configuration and contemplated fixation method.

A   Acute Valgus-Impacted Fractures

As the long head of the biceps is followed toward the rotator interval, the surgeon will encounter an osseous defect slightly posterior to the bicipital groove. This defect results from separation of the tuberosities as the head was crushed into valgus and

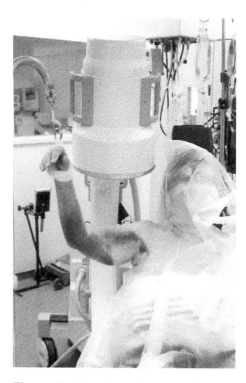

Figure 3 The C-arm is brought in from superiorly, parallel to the edge of the table. Anteroposterior and lateral views should be verified before preparing and draping the arm.

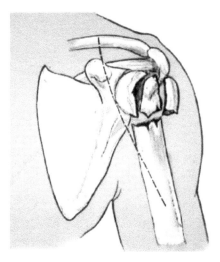

Figure 4 The skin incision parallels the deltopectoral interval and extends from slightly superior to the coracoid process toward the deltoid tuberosity.

impacted onto the humeral shaft. The periosteal sleeve between the tuberosities and the shaft will be intact; care should be taken not to disrupt it. A small periosteal elevator is placed through this osseous defect, and the head is tilted back into its normal anatomical position. A 2.5 mm terminally threaded pin is passed percutaneously through the deltoid to the anterolateral surface of the humeral shaft. The axillary nerve can be visualized on the deep surface of the deltoid so that the pin avoids it. The pin is driven in a retrograde fashion from the anterolateral shaft into the reduced head. The approximate angle of the pin is 45° in the coronal plane and 30° in the sagittal plane. Reduction and pin placement are verified by C-arm in both the anterior-posterior and axillary views. A second percutaneous pin is added, parallel to the first one.

The tuberosities are most often reduced anatomically or nearly anatomically with reduction of the head fragment. They are stabilized by interfragmentary nonabsorbable sutures crossed in the fracture site to prevent overreduction. Bone graft is usually not required in the acute setting. The pins are cut deep to the skin. Standard skin closure is performed.

B Subacute Valgus-Impacted Fractures

The humeral head fragment in subacute valgus-impacted four-part fractures has undergone early healing to the humeral shaft (Fig. 5A). The strength of the union between the humeral head and the shaft is a function of the elapsed time from injury. Moreover, the musculo-periosteal sleeve of tissue containing the tuberosities has begun to scar down into its shortened position, and periosteal new bone is beginning to form between this sleeve of tissue and the humeral shaft. All of these factors make reduction and stabilization more difficult than in the acute setting.

After identifying the long head of the biceps and following it proximally, the gap between the displaced tuberosities is identified. This will be more difficult than in the acute setting, but with careful dissection the defect can usually be found. Any soft tissue that has formed within the defect is excised so that the lateral margin of the head and the cancelleous surfaces of the tuberosities can be visualized (Fig. 5B). A small osteotome is driven carefully between the cancelleous undersurface of the head and the proximal humeral metaphysis. This is done very carefully and only a short distance at a time. The osteotome should not traverse the entire width of the humeral head as it might damage the inferomedial periosteal hinge. As the osteotome is advanced slowly across the humerus, it is gently levered superiorly so that the lateral aspect of the head is tilted back into its normal anatomical position (Fig. 5C). Provisional fixation can be obtained by placing a percutaneous pin through the deltoid and greater tuberosity into the head.

Depending on the elapsed time from injury, the tuberosities may not reduce anatomically. Should this occur, the periosteal sleeve is mobilized by shelling out some of the periosteal new bone. The tuberosities can then usually be reduced. Interfragmentary sutures are placed but not tied at this point.

In the subacute setting, the defect in the proximal humeral metaphysis left when the head is reduced is substantial. In addition, there is often a tendency for the head to collapse back into valgus. For these reasons, a blade-plate is used to support the head and cancellous allograft is packed between the top of the blade and the undersurface of the lateral portion of the head (Fig. 5D). The sequence of events is as follows. Cancelleous bone chips are packed under the reduced head through the gap in the tuberosities. The interfragmentary sutures between the tuberosities are tied. A malleable template is used to determine the length and contour of the plate. The guidewire from the blade-plate is placed 2–3 mm posterior to the bicipital groove approximately 2–3 cm distal to the tip of the greater tuberosity. The length of the blade is determined by measuring the guidewire, and an appropriate blade plate is chosen and contoured.

The C-arm is used to verify the reduction and guidewire placement before inserting the blade. The blade is then driven over the guidewire into the humeral metaphysis. Usually the blade enters the humerus at or near the original gap between the tuberosities. Consequently the bone is easily penetrated by the blade. The blade is driven up to the humeral head under C-arm guidance. Care is taken not to drive the blade too firmly into the head as this may result in splitting the head fragment or damage to the inferomedial periosteal hinge. At least three bicortical screws are

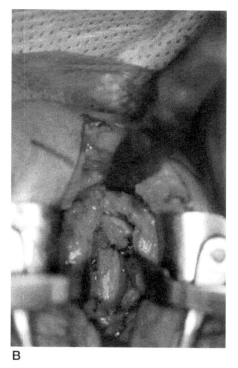

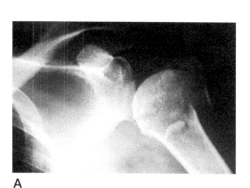

A   B

Figure 5 In a subacute valgus-impacted fracture, the impacted head has undergone early healing to the shaft (A). After the defect between the tuberosities has been identified, the lateral margin of the impacted head can be visualized through this defect (B). The head is reduced (elevated) with an elevator after an osteotome has recreated the fracture (C). A blade-plate is placed into the head through the defect in the tuberosities, and bone graft is inserted between the top of the blade and the inferior, cancelleous surface of the reduced head (D). An intraoperative image is taken to verify implant placement and head reduction (E). Postoperative radiographs demonstrate head reduction, implant placement, and bone graft placement (F).

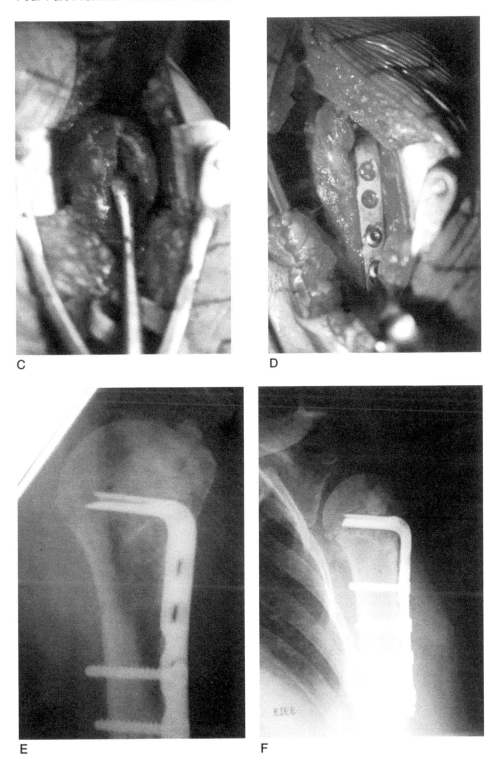

C   D

E   F

Figure 5 Continued.

placed through the plate into the humeral shaft. Additional bone graft is packed into the proximal humerus between the top of the blade and the head (Fig. 5E, F). Heavy nonabsorbable sutures are placed from the subscapularis, supraspinatus, infraspinatus tendons through the top hole in the plate. The provisional fixation pin is removed and a standard skin closure is accomplished.

C Standard Four-Part Fractures

A systematic approach to reduction and stabilization of standard four-part fractures is recommended (Fig. 6). Once the four fracture fragments have been identified, the head is aligned with the shaft and the greater tuberosity is reduced to the head fragment. Provisional fixation is obtained by placing a small k-wire from the greater tuberosity into the head and a second k-wire from the anterior aspect of the shaft (out of the way of the proposed area of placement of the plate) into the head. A cloverleaf plate contoured to the lateral cortex of the proximal humerus and with the superior and anterior leaves of the plate removed is placed on the anterolateral surface of the humerus. The plate is fixed to the distal fragment with one bicortical screw so that the top of the plate is approximately 1–2 cm from the top of the greater tuberosity.

The most superior screw in the plate is then placed. The hole should be drilled through the plate up to the subchondral bone using the C-arm to dictate depth. The hole should not be tapped, and a partially threaded cancelleous screw is utilized. This is the most important screw in the proximal fragment and should obtain enough purchase to bring the head and greater tuberosity directly up against the plate. The remaining screws in the proximal fragment are placed in a similar fashion. They should be angled to obtain maximum distance between each screw in the head. The remaining bicortical screws in the distal portion of the plate are placed. There should be a minimum of three bicortical screws in the distal fragment. The provisional fixation pins are removed.

The lesser tuberosity is reduced last, as described by Esser. It is held provisionally with a small k-wire. It is most easily stabilized to the greater tuberosity using interfragmentary sutures. Alternatively, a small interfragmentary screw can be used. The provisional fixation pin is removed and the final reduction and hardware position are verified using the C-arm. One fluoroscopic view while rotating the humerus will help exclude joint penetration by any of the screws. A standard skin closure is performed.

V PEARLS AND PITFALLS

Open reduction and internal fixation of four-part proximal humerus fractures is infrequently indicated and extremely difficult. In addition, multiple fixation options exist, and none has met with universal success. It is important to be prepared to use more than one fixation method. Moreover, if a reasonable reduction cannot be attained with stable enough fixation to allow early passive mobilization, prosthetic replacement may be the best option. Therefore, pearl number one—be prepared for anything!

The difference between one's visual impression of a fracture reduction and radiographic reality can be immense! Operative management of almost all proximal

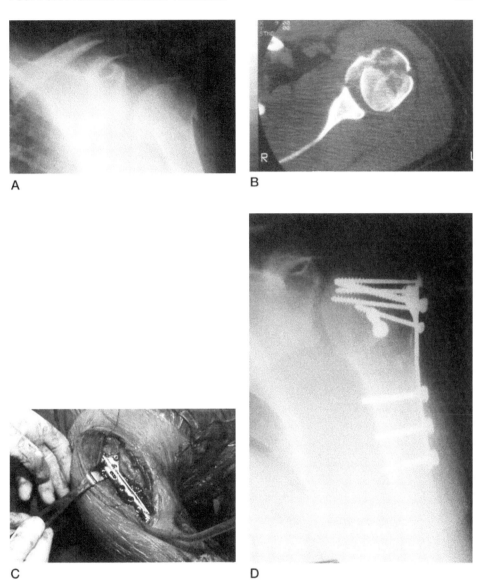

Figure 6 Anteroposterior radiograph (A) and CT scan (B) demonstrating a four-part fracture with a head-splitting component in a 27-year-old accident victim. Intraoperative picture demonstrating placement of a modified cloverleaf plate (C). Postoperative radiograph revealing adequate reduction and hardware placement (D). Radiograph taken 9 years postoperatively demonstrating avascular necrosis and posttraumatic arthritis (E). Clinical photograph demonstrating 9-year follow-up function. The patient is not symptomatic enough to require further treatment at this time (F). (Courtesy of Joseph Iannotti, MD, PhD.)

humerus fractures involves some element of indirect fracture reduction. The fragments are cloaked by the rotator cuff and glenohumeral joint capsule. It is much more desirable to become aware of a malreduction with the patient

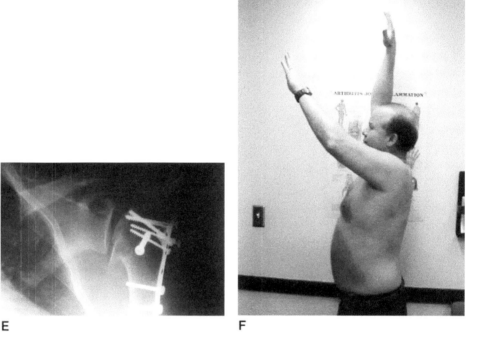

E   F

Figure 6   Continued.

anesthetized in the operating room than in the recovery room. Hence, pearl number two—use intraoperative radiographs or C-arm frequently.

It is unlikely that every fragment will be reduced anatomically on the first attempt. Even if two fragments are reduced adequately, the reduction may be lost when the remaining fragments are reduced or when additional hardware is placed. Furthermore, whatever reduction has been obtained must be verified radiographically. Pearl number three, therefore, is to use provisional fixation whenever possible.

The final pearl is to remember that the rotator cuff tendons are often stronger fixation points than the bone. Fixation obtained with any metallic fixation device can be reinforced with nonabsorbable sutures incorporating the rotator cuff tendons and the fracture fragments or plate. For example, the most proximal hole in a blade-plate is an excellent anchoring point for heavy nonabsorbable sutures passed through the tendon-bone junction of the rotator cuff.

Percutaneously placed pins can be a source of infection if left outside the skin. Often, pins protruding from the skin will drain. Oral antibiotics are ineffective in treating established pin tract infections. If the pin tract infection is not treated appropriately, chronic osteomyelitis may result (Fig. 7). Therefore, if a protruding pin begins to drain, it should be removed. Cutting the pins below the skin can prevent pin tract infections and the potential complication of osteomyelitis.

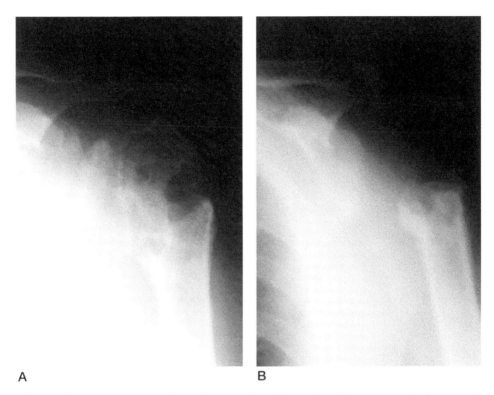

A   B

Figure 7 Percutaneous pins left protruding from the skin may result in chronic osteomyelitis and massive humeral head destruction (A). The destruction was severe enough in this patient to require humeral head resection (B).

VI POSTOPERATIVE REHABILITATION

In general, postoperative rehabilitation is similar in all types of operatively stabilized four-part fractures described above. Ideally, passive joint mobilization with pendulum exercises, supine passive flexion, and passive external rotation should begin on postoperative day 1. However, rehabilitation should be tailored according to the quality of fixation obtained. As a general rule, pendulum exercises begin within the first postoperative week. Radiographs are taken at the time of initial follow-up, which is usually within 7–10 days. If there is no displacement of the fracture and no hardware migration, supine passive flexion and external rotation commence. Another radiograph is taken at approximately 4–6 weeks postoperatively. If no problems are encountered, an overhead pulley is instituted. Passive stretching exercises within pain tolerance are instituted at 8–10 weeks postoperatively. Another radiograph is obtained 12 weeks postoperatively. If no radiographic signs of hardware failure or loss of reduction are identified, active, active assisted, and strengthening exercises are added and continue for 3–6 months. Final radiographic follow-up is obtained at 6 months postoperatively.

Percutaneously placed pins will cause irritation of the deltoid during rehabilitative exercises. The patient should be encouraged to perform the exercises within his or her pain tolerance. The pins can be removed at 3–4 weeks postoperatively; this will dramatically improve exercise tolerance. Other hardware such as plates and blade-plates do not require removal. However, if the patient develops symptoms from the hardware, such as subacromial impingement, the plate should not be removed for one year postoperatively unless radiographic union is absolutely certain. If the plate has been in for one year, there are no signs of hardware failure or loosening, the fracture reduction has not changed, and the fracture line(s) are not visible on routine radiography, fracture union is likely and the plate can be removed.

REFERENCES

1. Neer CS II. Displaced proximal humeral fractures part II. Treatment of three-part and four-part displacement. J Bone Joint Surg 1970; 52-A:1090–1103.
2. Hawkins RJ, Angelo RL. Displaced proximal humerus fractures. Selecting treatment, avoiding pitfalls. Orthop Clin North Am 1987; 18:421–431.
3. Compito CA, Self EB, Bigliani LU. Arthroplasty and acute shoulder trauma. Reasons for success and failure. Clin Orthop 1994; 307:27–36.
4. Resch H, Beck E, Bayley I. Reconstruction of the valgus-impacted humeral head fracture. J Shoulder Elbow Surg 1995; 4:73–80.
5. McLaughlin JA, Light R, Lustrin I. Axillary artery injury as a complication of proximal humerus fractures. J Shoulder Elbow Surg 1998; 7:292–294.
6. Jakob RP, Miniaci A, Anson PS, Jaberg H, Osterwalder A, Ganz R. Four-part valgus impacted fractures of the proximal humerus. J Bone Joint Surg 1991; 73-B:295–298.
7. Jaberg H, Warner JJP, Jakob RP. Percutaneous stabilization of unstable fractures of the humerus. J Bone Joint Surg 1992; 74-A:508–515.
8. Resch H, Povacz P, Fröhlich R, Wambacher M. Percutaneous fixation of three and four-part fractures of the proximal humerus. J Bone Joint Surg 1997; 79-B:295–300.
9. Mouradian WH. Displaced proximal humerus fractures. Seven years' experience with a modified Zickel supracondylar device. Clin Orthop 1986; 212:209–218.
10. Darder A, Darder A Jr, Sanchis V, Gastaldi E, Gomar F. Four-part displaced proximal humeral fractures: operative treatment using kirschner wires and a tension band. J Orthop Trauma 1993; 6:497–505.
11. Paavolainen P, Björkenheim JM, Slätis P, Paukku P. Operative treatment of severe proximal humeral fractures. Acta Orthop Scand 1983; 54:374–379.
12. Kristiansen B, Christensen SW. Plate fixation of proximal humeral fractures. Acta Orthop Scand 1986; 57:320–323.
13. Esser RD. Treatment of three and four-part fractures of the proximal humerus with a modified cloverleaf plate. J Orthop Trauma 1994; 8:15–22.
14. Szyszkowitz R, Seggl W, Schleifer P, Cundy PJ. Proximal humeral fractures. Management techniques and expected results. Clin Orthop 1993; 292:13–25.
15. Sehr JR, Szabo RM. Semitubular blade plate for fixation in the proximal humerus. J Orthop Trauma 1989; 2:327–332.
16. Zyto K, Ahrengart L, Sperber A, Törnkvist H. Treatment of displaced proximal humeral fractures in elderly patients. J Bone Joint Surg 1997; 79-B:412–417.

7

Humeral Head Replacement for Four-Part Proximal Humerus Fractures

ANAND M. MURTHI

University of Maryland School of Medicine, Baltimore, Maryland, U.S.A.

LOUIS U. BIGLIANI

Columbia University, College of Physicians and Surgeons, New York-Presbyterian Hospital, and Center for Shoulder, Elbow and Sports Medicine, New York, New York, U.S.A.

I INTRODUCTION

Prosthetic replacement of the humeral head for fracture remains an operative challenge to even the most experienced orthopedic surgeon. Although most fractures of the proximal humerus are minimally displaced and treated conservatively, more complex fractures require operative intervention. In this respect, the four-part proximal humerus fracture and fracture-dislocation have been difficult to evaluate and manage. Results from conservative treatment have been consistently unsatisfactory, while results from surgery have been more variable with some series reporting satisfactory results (1–7).

Treatment options for four-part fractures and fracture-dislocations of the proximal humerus fractures include nonoperative management, open reduction and internal fixation, and humeral head replacement (HHR). Nonoperative management of this complex fracture usually leads to poor results due to displacement of the fracture fragments and soft tissue adhesions. There is a high incidence of complications including osteonecrosis, malunion, nonunion, and degenerative glenohumeral disease (1). The functional disability resulting from conservative treatment of these fractures preclude this treatment option in active patients. Reports of the use of internal fixation have had variable results in the literature. These include metallic plates and screws, percutaneous pinning, and suture fixation with and without Enders rods. The poorest results are those attempted in the elderly and the best in those select young patients with valgus impacted fractures (2). An attempt may be made to preserve the native articular surface but the risks of avascular necrosis, malunion, nonunion, and revision surgeries are potential complications (2,8). However, to our knowledge no prospective comparison studies between internal fixation and hemiarthroplasty have been performed. Because of the poor results with nonoperative treatment, resection arthroplasty, and internal fixation, Neer in 1951 introduced prosthetic arthroplasty with tuberosity reconstruction for these complex fractures (3). Many reports in the literature have documented the successful results of this procedure (4,5,9,10). Prosthetic replacement of acute displaced fractures is technically demanding but offers a predictive result of a pain-free shoulder and functional motion through dedicated rehabilitation.

Our goals in this chapter are to provide stepwise, comprehensive information on the techniques and guidelines for HHR in the treatment of complex proximal humerus fractures. Careful preoperative planning, patient evaluation, imaging, meticulous operative techniques, and a closely supervised rehabilitation program are necessary to produce a successful functional shoulder after prosthetic reconstruction.

II INDICATIONS/PREOPERATIVE PLANNING

The indications for HHR for acute proximal humerus fractures are four-part fractures and fracture-dislocations, anatomical neck and head-splitting fractures that cannot be anatomically reduced and stabilized, and head impression fractures involving greater than 40% of the articular surface (11). Additionally, HHR is an alternative to open reduction and internal fixation for osteoporotic three-part fractures that occur in physiologically older, less active patients (6,12). In this situation the poor bone quality may not allow adequate stability with internal fixation to allow early motion.

Preoperative planning is critical before these complex reconstructions. First, a comprehensive history and physical must be performed to evaluate the patient's health status, associated injuries, comorbidities, fracture pattern, and ability to comply with strict rehabilitation. Of importance is a thorough documented preoperative neurovascular examination due to the significant incidence of brachial plexus neurapraxias and axillary artery injury. Elderly patients with atherosclerotic vessels may be at a higher risk of arterial damage with a proximal humerus fracture, especially in the face of significant ecchymoses and axillary swelling.

Next, proper imaging studies must be obtained for proper fracture classification. Standard trauma series anteroposterior, scapular lateral, and axillary radiographs will usually provide sufficient information necessary to identify fracture fragments, fracture displacement, and bone quality (Fig. 1A,B). On our service we prefer the Velpeau axillary view as the arm remains in the sling and painful manipulation of the injured shoulder is avoided (Fig. 1C). Also, rotational views may provide additional information regarding tuberosity displacement and angulation. However, in some select cases, computed tomography (CT) might provide additional information on comminution, articular surface damage, and tuberosity/shaft displacement in various planes (Fig. 2) (13).

The goal is to determine the position of the head with respect to the tuberosities, shaft, and glenoid. Next, it is critical to determine how many of the

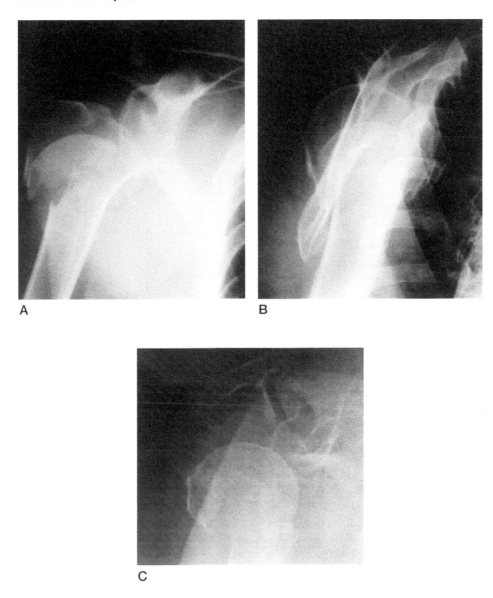

Figure 1 Standard trauma series (A) anteroposterior, (B) scapula lateral, and (C) Velpeau axillary radiographs.

tuberosities, if any, are attached to the head. Finally, assessment of articular damage to the humeral head and glenoid should be made. We also recommend templating the contralateral proximal humerus as a guide for choosing trial implants and

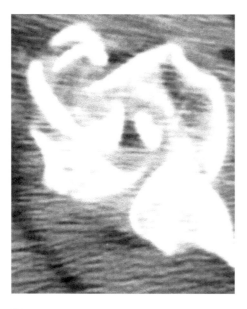

Figure 2 Computed tomography scan revealing four-part fracture of proximal humerus.

prostheses. Because most systems used modular components, efficiency and accuracy are crucial in selecting components when implanting the proper prosthesis.

Timing to surgery is also critical and should be performed as soon as the patient is medically stable, if possible within 7–10 days after the fracture. Delaying the surgery may be detrimental to exposure, inhibit tuberosity mobilization, cause capsular scarring and soft-tissue contractures, and increase the possibility of ectopic bone formation, thus diminishing postoperative functional motion. Healing of the tuberosities in a malunited position significantly increases the technical demands of this operation. Neer and McIlveen reported ectopic bone formation in 7 of 61 patients (16%) undergoing prosthetic replacement, and this complication usually occurred when surgery was delayed greater than 10 days (14). Surgical reconstruction in the early postinjury period is easier and allows more predictable outcomes (9).

III SURGICAL TECHNIQUE

Preoperatively, the shoulder and axilla should be kept hygienic and skin maceration should be avoided (e.g., in a tight sling). General or regional anesthesia may be used, but we prefer interscalene regional anesthesia because it is safe, effective, and allows excellent immediate postoperative analgesia. The patient is placed at the edge of the operative table in the modified beach-chair position with the head supported by a well-padded headrest. Placement of the operative shoulder over the lateral edge of the table allows for humeral extension and exposure during humeral canal preparation, reaming, and prosthetic insertion. Two folded towels are placed under the vertebral border of the scapula for lateral stabilization. A small arm-board is used at the level of the humeral shaft enabling the elbow and forearm to be supported during the initial exposure. This arm-board can then be shifted distally to allow for arm extension during humeral canal preparation. Then the shoulder is prepped and draped wide with the arm free to allow for positioning during surgery. Finally, iodine impregnated skin draping is placed to cover the operative site. Prophylactic broad-spectrum antibiotics are administered perioperatively for 24–48 hours.

A long deltopectoral approach is preferred for prosthetic replacement for a four-part fracture or fracture-dislocation. The coracoid process and deltoid tuberosity are identified and a skin incision is made just lateral to the coracoid extending towards the tuberosity for approximately 10–12 cm (Fig. 3). The deltopectoral interval is developed while preserving the origin of the deltoid and the cephalic vein. The superior 1–2 cm of the pectoralis major insertion may be released to enhance inferior exposure. Next, the coracoid and conjoined tendon are identified and the clavipectoral fascia is incised just lateral to these structures, taking care to protect the musculocutaneous nerve during medial retraction. The axillary nerve is palpated on the undersurface of the deltoid and must be protected during lateral retraction. The fascia has often been disrupted from the fracture, and the hematoma must be evacuated prior to identifying normal anatomy. Developing the subacromial and subdeltoid areas is important prior to fracture mobilization. An elevator is used to release adhesions from the undersurface of the acromion and in the subdeltoid region. Further exposure is achieved by abducting the arm to relax the deltoid. The hemorrhagic bursal tissue and hematoma must be irrigated and debrided. The leading edge of the coracoacromial ligament is excised to increase superior exposure (Fig. 4). Palpation of the subacromial space may reveal a prominent acromial spur, and an acromioplasty may be required. However, in our series of fracture patients, impingement is rarely a concomitant diagnosis, and we prefer to maintain the coracoacromial arch whenever possible for anterosuperior

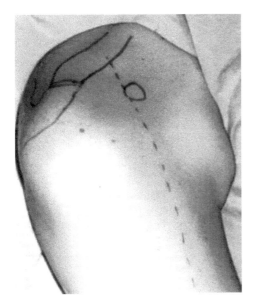

Figure 3   Long deltopectoral skin incision from the clavicle to the deltoid insertion.

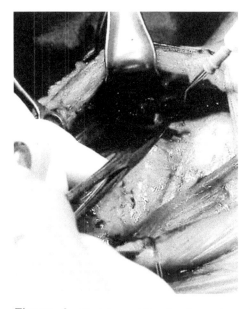

Figure 4 Excision of the leading edge of the coracoacromial ligament for superior exposure.

stability and function. Also, at this time the rotator cuff should be inspected for a rotator cuff tear. Acute or chronic rotator cuff tears are uncommon in patients with four-part fractures. Maintaining the coracoacromial arch should preserve its buffering function, thus preventing future superior humeral head migration.

Identifying the fracture segments and meticulous handling of comminuted fragments is important. Care must be taken in identifying the long head of the biceps tendon, following it proximally into the rotator interval between the lesser and greater tuberosities. Since the bicipital groove is often involved in the fracture, the tendon should be identified just underneath the leading edge of the pectoralis major insertion (Fig. 5). The greater tuberosity is usually displaced posteriorly and superiorly (underneath the acromion) because of the unopposed pull of the supraspinatus and infraspinatus muscles. The greater tuberosity is often displaced so far posterior that head removal must be performed prior to its identification and mobilization. The lesser tuberosity is displaced medially by the pull of the subscapularis muscle. It may be situated medially under the coracoid muscles, and care must be taken to avoid injury to the neurovascular structures during dissection.

Next, heavy nonabsorbable (number 2 and 5) nylon sutures with swedged-on needles are placed through the bone tendon junction of both tuberosities for traction (Fig. 6). This facilitates mobilization of the tuberosities with their rotator cuff attachments. Attempts at passing suture needles through bone may cause further comminution and bone loss as elderly patients often have significant osteoporosis. Once this is completed, further evaluation of additional fracture lines must be performed to prevent disruption of their soft tissue envelopes, which will assist in healing. Moreover, during mobilization of the lesser tuberosity, care must be taken

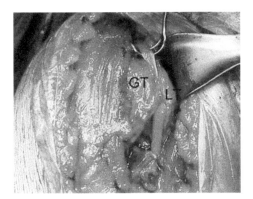

Figure 5 The long head of the biceps tendon (BT) identifies the interval between the lesser (LT) and greater tuberosities (GT).

to protect the circumflex vessels as well as the axillary nerve on its inferior border as these may be entrapped or scarred in the fracture site if surgery has been delayed.

Next, the rotator interval may be extended towards the coracoid to gain exposure and retrieve the humeral head (Fig. 7). The long head of the biceps tendon is a useful guide in this dissection. However, in cases where the interval and tuberosities are attached in their soft tissue sleeve, this may be maintained. They may be elevated together as a hood for access to the humeral head. In fracture-dislocations care must be taken to atraumatically retrieve the humeral head. It is usually intracapsular underneath the subscapularis tendon, but it may be extracapsular and adjacent to the neurovascular bundle. Therefore, if preoperative x-rays reveal a medially and inferiorly displaced humeral head deep in the axilla, care must be taken as sharp fragment edges may injure the close neurovascular structures. Vascular clamps and at least two units of patient-specific blood should be available at all times. If the head is scarred in posteriorly it may require an osteotomy to be

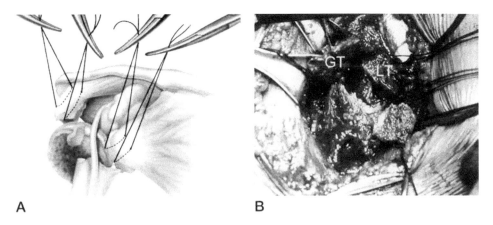

A   B

Figure 6 (A and B) Sutures are placed at the bone-tendon junction while mobilizing the lesser (LT) and greater tuberosities (GT).

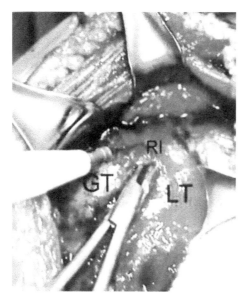

Figure 7 Extension of the rotator interval (RI) allows exposure to the articular surface.

removed in piecemeal fashion. The head should be saved for a potential source of cancellous bone graft to augment the tuberosity reconstruction to the prosthesis. The graft may be placed in either a doughnut configuration, U-shape, or multiple pieces placed underneath and alongside the tuberosity reconstruction. The amount of bone used depends on the amount of bone left on the tuberosities and the proximal shaft. The long head of the biceps tendon is retracted posterolaterally during preparation of the humerus.

Preparation of the humerus must be performed with the arm in extension, adduction, and external rotation to deliver the shaft into the operative field and protect the axillary nerve. Sequential reaming is performed until a cortical bite is obtained, then provisional stems are used to optimize the humeral fit. Preoperative templating may assist in choosing the correct size humeral stem. We routinely use cement fixation in our fracture prostheses due to osteopenic bone in the elderly population and to gain immediate height and rotational stability. There is no need to obtain a press-fit reduction of the humeral stem into the canal and too large a stem *and* cement increases the risk of intraoperative humeral shaft fracture and its associated complications.

Correct retroversion of the prosthetic stem remains crucial for final component stability and function. First, identification of the usual landmarks to obtain normal retroversion in the range of 30–40° should be performed. The prosthetic head should be retroverted in relation to the epicondylar axis of the distal humerus. Also, placing the fin of the prosthesis approximately 3–5 mm posterior and medial to the bicipital groove should offer the proper degree of version and lateral humeral offset (Fig. 8). In addition, with our system, alignment rods (Zimmer, Warsaw, IN) provide a further check for appropriate version between 20 and 40 degrees (Fig. 9). The surgeon should compare the stability of the construct based on the soft tissue and

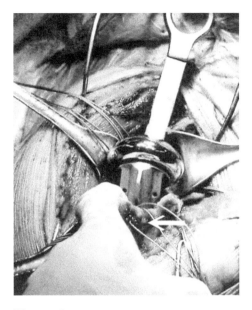

Figure 8 The prosthetic fin should be placed just posterior and medial to the bicipital groove (white arrow) to obtain proper version.

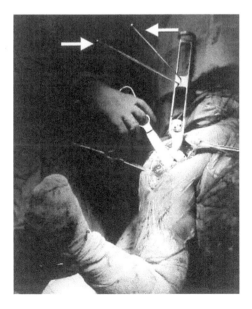

Figure 9 Alignment rods (white arrows) allow accurate version to be obtained. (Courtesy of Zimmer, Warsaw, IN.)

bony architecture. Previous techniques advocated to neutral (0°) version in posterior dislocations, but we have found this to be problematic leading to anterior instability. Therefore, we recommend less retroversion (~ 10–20°) for posterior fracture-dislocations and more retroversion for anterior fracture-dislocations.

The native head initially determines proper head size, and it should be measured after removal (Fig. 10). Another useful technique is using an AP x-ray of the contralateral shoulder as a template. Trial reductions using modular prosthetic components (Zimmer, Warsaw, IN) to test for longitudinal and rotational stability is important. A sponge placed down the shaft will stabilize the stem to allow stable manipulation (Fig. 11). Men tend to require a larger head size. Proper fit should allow maximum motion with stability in both the anteroposterior and superoinferior planes. There should be approximately 50% translation in both directions. There should be at least 45° external rotation without anterior dislocation of the head. The correct head size should allow closure of the tuberosities and rotator interval without tension on the repair. When deciding between head sizes it is usually better to select the smaller head as this will facilitate motion. A smaller head occupies less capsular volume and allows further excursion of the posteroinferior capsule required for arm extension. Also, a smaller prosthetic head facilitates tuberosity reattachment. Therefore, using modular implants will allow the surgeon to decide which size offers the most motion with stability. By reducing the tuberosities to the trial prosthesis with the previously placed traction sutures, the stability of the construct may be tested.

Obtaining proper prosthetic height is crucial in maintaining adequate tension in the myofascial sleeve and deltoid function and prevents postoperative impingement. Prior to trial stem placement, comminution of the proximal shaft must be stabilized with cerclage wires or sutures to provide optimum stability of the

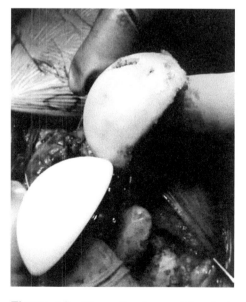

Figure 10 The native humeral head should be measured against potential sizes for replacement. (Courtesy of Zimmer, Warsaw, IN.)

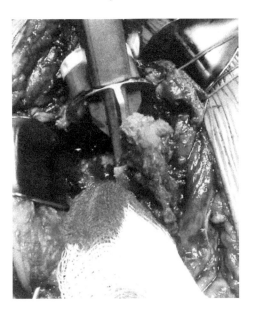

Figure 11   A sponge placed down the shaft allows proper humeral height to be tested.

prosthesis and prevent subsidence. As mentioned previously, placement of a sponge down the shaft supports the trial stem and provides an accurate guide to height (Fig. 11). The greater tuberosity should just overlap the proximal shaft cortex, and the inferior hole on the prosthetic fin should remain just above the proximal cortical margin of the humeral shaft. Stability at the proper height should allow 50% translation with the push-pull test in both the anteroposterior and superoinferior planes.

Placement of the prosthesis below the anticipated greater tuberosity site may cause impingement as well as a lax soft tissue envelope, resulting in glenohumeral instability. On the other hand, placing the stem too proud effectively decreases the space under the coracoacromial arch and will lead to postoperative stiffness and impaired motion. It may also impinge against the native glenoid. The tension in the biceps tendon as it courses over the prosthetic head may provide assistance as a marker of proper stem height. If there is a gap between the humeral shaft and head, pieces of corticocancellous graft from the humeral head may be used to support the prosthesis at the correct height. The trial humeral stem and head should be reduced on the glenoid to assess internal and external rotation. If the construct is stable to 40–50°, external rotation and internal rotation at the side then the retroversion is appropriate.

Prior to cementing the stem, multiple drill holes are made in the humeral shaft for attachment of the tuberosities. Nonabsorbable number 2 or 5 sutures are placed through these holes, using 3–4 sutures for the greater tuberosity and 2–3 sutures for the lesser tuberosity fragments (Fig. 12). These sutures are reduction sutures to fix the tuberosities to the humeral shaft below the prosthetic head. Cement is placed in the humeral shaft, and the prosthesis is placed in the proper position and held

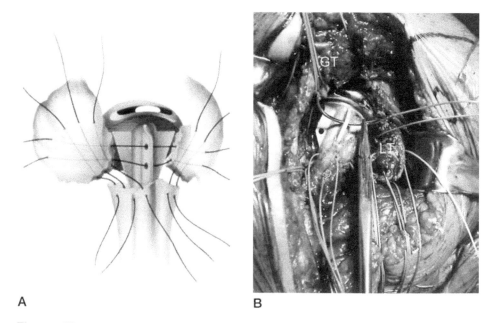

A   B

Figure 12   (A and B) Sutures are placed through the greater (GT) and lesser (LT) tuberosities, prosthetic fin, and humeral shaft for reconstruction.

until the cement is firm. We recommend removing the most proximal cement prior to hardening and placing bone graft to facilitate tuberosity healing. A cement restrictor should be used to avoid distal runoff of cement down the shaft. Importantly, one must avoid pressurizing the canal with doughy cement as osteoporotic bone may easily fracture.

After the humeral stem has been cemented, focus turns to reconstructing the tuberosities and their associated rotator cuff attachments. First, the biceps tendon is relocated within its groove and the rotator interval. Then, using the previously placed sutures in the tuberosities and shaft, the tuberosities are reduced to the proximal humeral shaft, prosthetic fin, and each other (Fig. 12B). First, the greater tuberosity is reduced, followed by the lesser tuberosity. The more posterior sutures are tied first. Then the lesser tuberosity sutures are tied down to the shaft. Finally, the two transverse sutures through the fins of the prosthesis, and both tuberosities are tied down to promote compression of the tuberosities to the shaft, bone graft, and prosthesis. The transverse sutures should be placed prior to tying down the tuberosity to shaft sutures. Of importance is placement of the tuberosities (especially the greater) below the level of the prosthetic head to prevent postoperative impingement. Recent interest has centered on circlage sutures around the neck of the prosthesis as an adjuvant technique in tuberosity reconstruction. This may be a useful technique, as is a criss-cross technique of tuberosity to shaft fixation from the greater tuberosity to the medial shaft and the lesser tuberosity to the lateral shaft. However, it should be pointed out that tuberosity to shaft fixation (and healing) is critical to the success of this operation. If the tuberosities are not adequately repaired to the shaft (and heal to the shaft), then this procedure will fail. Finally, only the lateral aspect of the rotator interval is reapproximated (Fig. 13). Medial closure of the rotator interval will significantly diminish external rotation. The previously incised pectoralis major tendon insertion is reapproximated to the humeral shaft.

The final evaluation involves taking the arm through a gentle limited range of motion while inspecting for prosthetic impingement and tuberosity fixation to the components and shaft. Intraoperative radiographs or fluoroscopy (if necessary) will reveal if the position of the prosthesis and tuberosities are adequately aligned. Next, hemovac drains are placed deep to the deltoid and the incision is closed in layers with a final subcuticular closure. The limb is immobilized postoperatively in a well-padded sling and swathe with the arm in a neutral position at the side. It is important to avoid the Velpeau position postoperatively as this may lead to posterior subluxation or dislocation.

IV REHABILITATION

Carefully monitored postoperative rehabilitation remains crucial to obtaining a good functional result. The patient must understand the phases and restrictions of rehabilitation and the goals must be realistic both for the surgeon and patient. The three-phase system of Hughes and Neer is our protocol and is individualized per patient depending on a variety of factors (15).

Depending on the strength of surgical repair and the preoperative and intraoperative assessment of bone and soft tissue quality the rehabilitation protocol is modified. Factors to consider are the status of the rotator cuff, stability of the

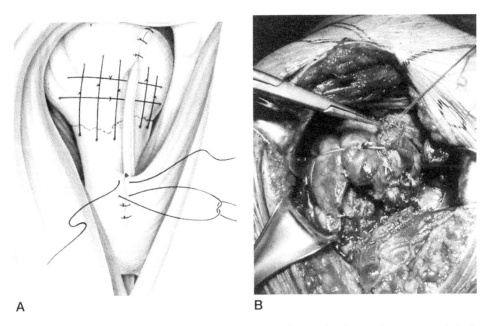

A   B

Figure 13 (A and B) Tuberosities must be repaired to each other and the proximal shaft below the level of the prosthetic head. The rotator interval (clamp) is closed.

tuberosity reconstruction, extent of comminution, use of bone graft, and the ability of the patient to participate in supervised physical therapy. The surgeon should gently range the shoulder after reconstruction to determine the safe zone of motion.

The arm is supported in a sling, and an axillary pad is helpful in the early postoperative period. Active hand and elbow motion is allowed. The first goal is to reestablish glenohumeral and scapulothoracic motion. Passive motion is started on the first postoperative day with the therapist teaching and assisting with elevation to approximately 80–90° along with gentle gravity-assisted pendulum exercises. Supine passive external rotation, within the limits of surgery, is started using the opposite arm or a stick. Avoid pulley-assisted elevation until the tuberosities are healed as these exercises involve a significant active component. The patient needs to be reassured often but must be warned that overly aggressive early active motion will result in tuberosity detachment and possible dislocation (16).

Exercises should be performed three times daily under the direct supervision of a therapist until discharge. Patients should exercise independently as soon as they can perform them in a safe manner. Friends or family members involved with care should be taught to assist the patient in their rehabilitation. At hospital discharge, patients should reach approximately 130–140° elevation and 20–30° external rotation at the side. These passive exercises should be continued for approximately 6 weeks or until radiographic evidence of tuberosity healing.

Active-assisted motion with the contralateral arm and pulleys along with isometric strengthening of the deltoid and rotator cuff are started after evidence of tuberosity healing (usually 6–8 weeks). Next, progressive strengthening and resistive exercises are added to the regimen over a 2- to 3-week period. Gradually the patient is taught to use the operative arm more and withdraw assistance from the contralateral arm during therapy. Shoulder extension and internal rotation stretching exercises are now instituted. Patients are allowed and encouraged to perform activities of daily living. More aggressive stretching and strengthening is started approximately 12 weeks postoperatively. Theraband resistance exercises and light weights are begun when the patient is pain-free and has achieved almost complete motion. Finally, gentle stretching and strengthening should be included in the daily protocol and patients should continue their regimen from 6 months to one year to obtain maximum results and function. It is important to use these recommendations as guidelines in postoperative therapy as each patient might not reach these goals or may need to accelerate or temper their rehabilitation.

V RADIOGRAPHIC FOLLOW-UP

Radiographs of the prosthetic replacement should be obtained immediately postoperatively and after physical therapy has been initiated. Any evidence of tuberosity malposition or displacement after therapy should be corrected for functional results to be optimal. After discharge patients should be followed closely with sequential radiographs before progressing to active exercises in therapy. Evidence of tuberosity healing is important prior to advancing therapy. Thereafter, radiographs at 6 months and then yearly should be obtained to monitor for prosthesis/tuberosity position, glenoid wear, osteolysis, stem subsidence, and loosening.

VI   AVOIDING COMPLICATIONS

Complications are not uncommon in these complex reconstructions and are usually the result of inadequate technique or lack of patient compliance with postoperative instructions regarding rehabilitation (16).

A   Tuberosity Malposition/Nonunion/Malunion

Malposition of the tuberosities usually involves the greater tuberosity with its posterior rotator cuff insertion. This is a significant complication. Greater tuberosity displacement and malunion creates a problem with strength and motion postoperatively. Also, patients with osteopenic bone may develop this problem as fixation may fail and delay healing. Posterior tuberosity displacement blocks motion and weakens external rotation, while superior displacement into the subacromial space causes impingement and is a mechanical block to elevation and abduction. Lesser tuberosity displacement is medial and may block and weaken internal rotation. Also loss of the lesser tuberosity fixation may lead to anterior dislocation and difficulty in initiating forward elevation. Therefore it is of great importance to focus on tuberosity fixation to the shaft, prosthetic fin, and each other. Multiple, heavy, nonabsorbable sutures at the bone tendon junction are the key in this part of the reconstruction. Stressing that the tuberosities heal to the shaft and each other and not the prosthesis is important. Local bone graft is often needed to bridge the gap between the tuberosities and shaft and provides stability. Any signs of early displacement should be treated with revision tuberosity repair. Of utmost importance is preventing active motion for at least 6 weeks to prevent tuberosity pull off from rotator cuff contraction. Furthermore, evidence of tuberosity nonunion with displacement leading to pain and poor shoulder function is a relative indication for revision surgery and tuberosity reconstruction with the possibility of iliac crest bone grafting (7).

B   Prosthetic Loosening

Humeral loosening, while rare, may occur in those patients with proximal shaft comminution and osteopenia. Cement fixation, therefore, is essential to minimize this risk. Serial radiographic monitoring for loosening and correct positioning are important aspects of initial evaluation. If prosthesis loosening occurs despite adequate cement fixation, then evaluation for signs of infection should be considered.

C   Prosthetic Malposition

Component malposition usually involves improper version, height, or head size. First, improper version may result in anterior or posterior instability and/or decreased motion from an incongruent glenohumeral joint. Guidelines to impart correct version include the following:

1.   The prosthetic fin should be placed approximately 5 mm posteromedial to the bicipital groove.
2.   Palpating the distal humeral epicondylar axis to keep the arm in neutral rotation gives a guide to approximating 20–40°.

3. Using alignment rods that attach to the humeral insertion device provides a choice between 20 and 40° retroversion of the humeral head.
4. While holding the elbow flexed at 90° and the arm in neutral rotation, the prosthetic head should point towards the glenoid.
5. The prosthesis should remain stable during functional internal and external rotation.

Next, prosthesis height is important in preventing greater tuberosity impingement by being seated too low. Also, there may be inferior instability secondary to a lax myofascial sleeve. A proud stem may effectively "overstuff" the subacromial space and lead to stiffness. The key is to produce a humerotuberal interval intraoperatively of approximately 5 mm. The greater tuberosity must remain below the humeral head while maintaining adequate tension in the rotator cuff and deltoid.

D Postoperative Stiffness

Achieving and maintaining motion is foremost for a successful outcome after humeral head replacement. Meticulous operative technique, secure tuberosity/prosthesis fixation, and early postoperative supervised motion are all important in obtaining full range of motion. We cannot overly stress the importance of patient compliance with early rehabilitation (15). It is important to obtain early passive functional motion, as it is very difficult to increase motion after the initial passive phase of exercises.

VII CASE ILLUSTRATION

A 65-year-old right hand–dominant man tripped and fell on his outstretched right arm. He complained of severe pain and swelling in his right shoulder only. On physical examination the right shoulder was markedly swollen and ecchymosed and his neurovascular examination was within normal limits. Radiographs revealed a comminuted four-part fracture of the proximal humerus. Two days following his injury he underwent a cemented humeral head replacement and tuberosity reconstruction without complication. Postoperative films show proper fixation of the greater and lesser tuberosities below the humeral head and maintenance of the humerotuberal interval (Fig. 14). Radiographs after 6 weeks revealed healing of the tuberosities, and he was allowed to being the active strengthening portion of rehabilitation. At one year he was pain-free and able to perform most activities of daily living and had active elevation to 165° and external rotation to 40° at the side. He was very satisfied with his result.

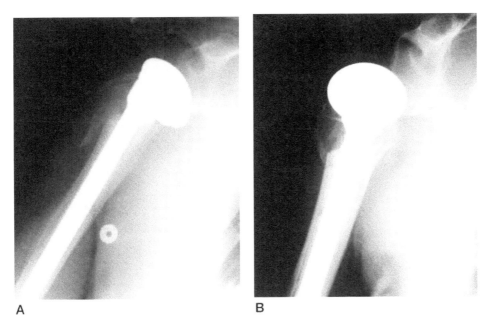

A   B

Figure 14 (A and B) Postoperative radiographs revealed tuberosity fixation below the prosthetic head retaining the humerotuberal interval.

REFERENCES

1. Stableforth PG. Four-part fractures of the neck of the humerus. J Bone Joint Surg (Br) 1984; 66(1):104–108.
2. Resch H, Beck E, Bayley I. Reconstruction of the valgus-impacted humeral head fracture. J Shoulder Elbow Surg 1995; 4(2):73–80.
3. Neer CSI. Articular replacement for the humeral head. J Bone Joint Surg (Am) 1955; 37A:215–228.
4. Green A, Barnard L, Limbird RS. Humeral head replacement for acute, four-part proximal humerus fractures. J Shoulder Elbow Surg 1993; 2:249–254.
5. Goldman RT, Koval KJ, Cuomo F, Gallagher MA, Zuckerman JD. Functional outcome after humeral head replacement for acute three- and four-part proximal humeral fractures. J Shoulder Elbow Surg 1995; 4(2):81–86.
6. Zyto K, Wallace WA, Frostick SP, Preston BJ. Outcome after hemiarthroplasty for three- and four-part fractures of the proximal humerus. J Shoulder Elbow Surg 1998; 7(2):85–89.
7. Tanner MW, Cofield RH. Prosthetic arthroplasty for fractures and fracture-dislocations of the proximal humerus. Clin Orthop 1983; 179:116–128.
8. Bigliani LU. Malunion of four-part anterior fracture-dislocation following open reduction internal fixation. Tech Orthop 1994; 9(2):99–101.
9. Neer CSI. Fractures. In: Shoulder Reconstruction. Philadelphia: WB Saunders, 1990:363–420.
10. Moeckel BH, Dines DM, Warren RF, Altchek DW. Modular hemiarthroplasty for fractures of the proximal part of the humerus. J Bone Joint Surg (Am) 1992; 74(6):884–889.

11. Bigliani LU, Flatow EL, Pollock RG. The shoulder. In: Rockwood CA, Master FAI, eds. The Shoulder. Philadelphia: WB Saunders, 1998:337–374.

12. Cofield RH. Comminuted fractures of the proximal humerus. Clin Orthop 1988; 230:49–57.

13. Sjoden GO, Movin T, Guntner P, Aspelin P, Ahrengart L, Ersmark H, Sperber A. Poor reproducibility of classification of proximal humeral fractures. Additional CT of minor value. Acta Orthop Scand 1997; 68(3):239–242.

14. Neer CSI. Recent results and techniques of prosthetic replacement for 4-part proximal humeral fractures. Orthop Trans 1986; 10:475.

15. Hughes M, Neer CS. Glenohumeral joint replacement and postoperative rehabilitation. Phys Ther 1975; 55(8):850–858.

16. Bigliani LU, Flatow EL, McCluskey GW, Fischer RA. Failed prosthetic replacement in dsiplaced proximal humerus fractures. Orthop Trans 1991; 15:747–748.

8

Arthroscopically Assisted Open Reduction and Internal Fixation of Proximal Humerus Fractures

CHRISTOPHER K. JONES

Southern Orthopedics/Sports Medicine, La Grange, Georgia, U.S.A.

FELIX H. SAVOIE III

Mississippi Sports Medicine and Orthopedic Center, Jackson, Mississippi, U.S.A.

I INTRODUCTION

Fractures of the proximal humerus are relatively common and account for 4–5% of all fractures (1–3). The vast majority of these fractures (85%) are minimally displaced and are adequately managed nonoperatively with immobilization followed by early motion. The remaining 15% of these fractures are displaced. The functional outcome of treating displaced fractures nonoperatively is suboptimal, and some form of reduction and fixation is indicated (1,4). However, there is considerable disagreement with regard to classification of these fractures, the indications for surgical management, the surgical approach, and the method of fixation.

There are reports of the arthroscope being used to assist in reduction of articular fractures of the scaphoid, distal radius, the proximal tibia, and the glenoid (5–12). We are unaware, however, of any published reports of arthroscopically assisted open reduction and internal fixation of proximal humerus fractures.

We have used an arthroscopically assisted approach to open reduction and internal fixation of certain types of fractures of the proximal humerus. We have found that glenohumeral and subacromial arthroscopy allow reduction of the fracture fragments and fixation with a limited open exposure.

II INDICATIONS/CONTRAINDICATIONS

Although several studies have demonstrated poor intra- and interobserver reliability of the four-part classification reported by Neer, it remains the standard classification of proximal humerus fractures (2,13,14). As detailed in Chapter 1, a part is considered displaced if it is displaced 1 cm or angulated 45 degrees. Surgery is indicated for fractures that meet these criteria for displacement.

Recently, several authors have questioned these criteria for displacement of greater tuberosity fractures. They stress that greater tuberosity fractures with greater than 5 mm of displacement can lead to primary impingement and loss of external rotation if reduction is not accomplished (15). The managing physician must differentiate high-velocity from low-velocity fractures of the tuberosity. Low-velocity fractures often occur in the elderly during a fall. The tuberosity is levered off by the acromion as the arm abducts. These patients will have minimally displaced fractures with little collateral damage. When displaced, reduction and fixation is easily accomplished in the acute setting.

Young patients may sustain an injury that appears radiographically similar to these low-velocity injuries. However, in these patients the shoulder dislocates, tearing the capsule and/or labrum (Fig. 1). The arm continues to rotate and the tuberosity is forced off, pulling apart the rotator interval (Fig. 2) and rotator cuff, in addition to the greater tuberosity fracture.

We have used the arthroscope to assist in the reduction and fixation of greater and lesser tuberosity fractures, as well as some head splitting fractures. The arthroscope aids in obtaining an accurate reduction of the fragments and also allows for assessment of the rotator cuff and intra-articular pathology. We have found that a high percentage of patients with displaced tuberosity fractures will have an associated rotator cuff tear, rotator interval tear, and/or a capsulolabral tear, depending on age and mechanism of injury as listed above.

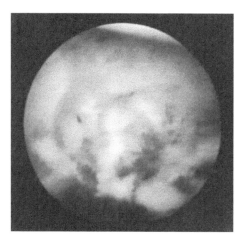

Figure 1 Anterior labral avulsion in patient with greater tuberosity fracture.

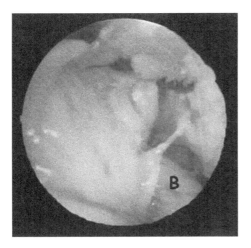

Figure 2 Rotator interval tear in patient with greater tuberosity fracture (B = biceps tendon).

III PREOPERATIVE PLANNING

The preoperative planning stage consists of a thorough history, physical examination, and radiographic evaluation. The history should focus on determining if any comorbidities exist that would preclude the patient from being a surgical candidate. The physical examination should consist of a detailed secondary survey to assess for any associated injuries. It should also include a detailed neurovascular examination. Special attention should be directed toward assessing the axillary nerve, as it is the most commonly injured nerve with proximal humerus fractures (1).

Radiographic exam should include the minimum of three views, which constitute the "trauma series." These include a true anterior-posterior view (Fig. 3A), a scapular view (Fig. 3B), and an axillary view. These three views are necessary

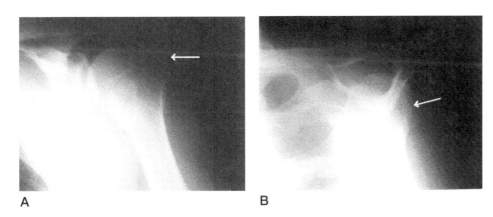

A   B

Figure 3 (A) Radiographic anterior-posterior view of greater tuberosity fracture. (B) Radiographic scapular view of greater tuberosity fracture.

in order to properly assess and classify the fracture pattern and to assess for an associated glenohumeral dislocation.

A computed tomography (CT) scan is obtained if there is a question regarding the degree of displacement or if the fracture pattern cannot be adequately assessed with plain radiographs. It is unusual to need a CT scan if well-done plain radiographs are obtained.

Attempted closed reduction of greater tuberosity fractures that are displaced more than 5 mm is done by placing the arm in an abduction sling with the shoulder externally rotated. If reduction is not adequate, consideration for arthroscopically assisted reduction and internal fixation is given. Continued displacement of 5 mm or more is an indication for repair.

IV   OPERATIVE APPROACHES

Traditionally, these fractures have been managed with an open approach and internal fixation with a variety of constructs. Two-part lesser tuberosity fractures, three-part lesser tuberosity fractures, four-part fractures, and two-part surgical neck fractures are usually approached through the deltopectoral interval, while for two-part greater tuberosity fractures, a superior deltoid splitting approach is utilized.

More recently, attempts to minimize surgical morbidity and the risk of avascular necrosis have led to the development of closed reduction and percutaneous fixation techniques for unstable two- and three-part fractures (16,17). These authors did not treat severely displaced, irreducible fractures or fractures that involved splitting of the articular surface.

An arthroscopically assisted reduction and fixation offers advantages over the traditional open approach to these fractures. The arthroscope allows for reduction of displaced fragments under direct visualization, while fixation can be performed through a percutaneous approach. This precludes the need for the extensive dissection that is required for the deltoid splitting approach. With less dissection in the subdeltoid space, there is less scarring and fewer problems with regaining motion postoperatively. Additionally, postoperative pain is diminished and patients will require less hospitalization and narcotics. The arthroscope also allows for assessment and treatment of concomitant intra-articular pathology.

The disadvantages of the arthroscopically assisted treatment of these fractures include its technical difficulty in visualizing, accurately assessing, and treating them through the arthroscope. A high level of skill and experience with shoulder arthroscopy is needed to attain a desirable outcome.

V   MY PERSONAL APPROACH

After general anesthesia is administered, the patient is positioned in the lateral decubitus position. A careful examination under anesthesia is performed to evaluate for any occult instability or loss of motion. The shoulder and upper extremity are prepped and draped. The arm is then placed in longitudinal traction with 10 pounds.

A diagnostic arthroscopy is performed and any coexisting intra-articular pathology is addressed. If a Bankart lesion is present, this is repaired prior to reduction and fixation of the fracture. The scope is placed into the subacromial space from the posterior portal and bursectomy is performed by a shaver introduced

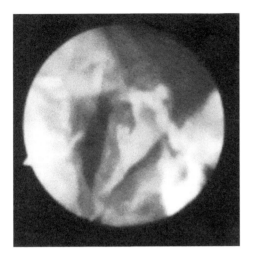

Figure 4 Bony bed for greater tuberosity fracture.

through a lateral portal. The fracture is visualized and its bony bed is debrided (Fig. 4). A reduction is performed while visualizing the fracture fragment through the scope. A probe can be inserted via the lateral portal to manipulate the fragment. If necessary, the arthroscope can be moved to the lateral or anterior portal in order to get another perspective of the fracture. A guide wire for a 4.5 or 6.5 mm cannulated screw is placed across the fracture towards the medial surgical neck (Fig. 5). This can be inserted directly through the skin at the lateral margin of the acromion. Quality of the reduction and position of the guide wire is assessed fluoroscopically. A second guide wire is always placed in order to prevent rotation of the fragment (Fig. 6). Two

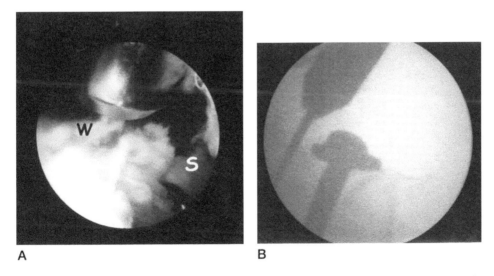

A   B

Figure 5 Screw and wire: (A) scope view; (B) radiographic view (W = wire, S = screw).

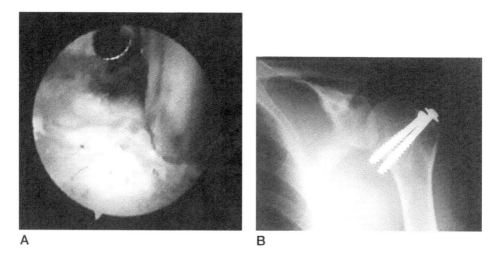

Figure 6   Final fixation: (A) scope view; (B) radiographic view.

screws are placed. A washer is preferred on both screws because of the tendency for the tuberosity bone to be soft.

After the fracture is internally fixed, the rotator cuff is carefully assessed for an interval tear. If a tear is present, it can be repaired using arthroscopic techniques.

VI   PEARLS AND PITFALLS

1. Watch out for bursal covering of cuff tear.
2. Greater tuberosity displaces posteriorly and medially.
3. Look for labral tear.
4. Repair rotator interval.
5. Check motion—acromioplasty often is beneficial if screw head is prominent.

VII   POSTOPERATIVE MANAGEMENT

The patient is placed in an abduction sling for 4 weeks. Passive mobilization is initiated in the first week. Active motion is delayed until healing is noted, usually 4–6 weeks.

VIII   REHABILITATION

The postoperative rehabilitation program must be individualized based on the fracture pattern and stability of fixation. Patients are typically immobilized in a sling for comfort, but passive mobilization is started as soon as tolerated. We begin with simple pendulum exercises and gentle passive range of motion. If percutaneous fixation has been performed, the pins are typically removed after 4 weeks. After approximately 8 weeks, when clinical and radiographic union has occurred, we begin gentle active motion and stretching. Once the patient has obtained a full active range of motion, resistive exercises are initiated.

IX RADIOGRAPHS

Radiographs are performed at the first postoperative visit to assess hardware position. We repeat them again at approximately 6–8 weeks postoperatively in order to assess healing. If clinical healing progresses as expected, repeat radiographs are not performed.

REFERENCES

1. Williams GR, Wong KL. Two and three part fractures: open reduction and internal fixation versus closed reduction and percutaneous pinning. Orthop Clin North Am 2000; 3(1):1–21.
2. Horak J, Nilsson BE. Epidemiology of fractures of the upper end of the humerus. CORR 1975; 112:250–253.
3. Rose SH, Melton LJ, Morrey BF, et al. Epidemiologic features of humeral fractures. CORR 1982; 168:24.
4. Wright JM, Hawkins RJ. Three-part fractures of the proximal humerus: technique of open reduction and internal fixation with tension-band wire. Tech Shoulder Elbow Surg 2000; 11:9–17.
5. Toh S, Nagao A, Harata S. Severely displaced scaphoid fracture treated by arthroscopic assisted reduction and osteosynthesis. J Orthop Trauma 2000; 14(4):299–302.
6. Taras JS, Sweet S, Shum W, et al. Percutaneous and arthroscopic screw fixation of scaphoid fractures. Hand Clin 1999; 15(3):467–473.
7. Doi K, Hattori Y, Otsuka K, et al. Intra-articular fractures of the distal aspect of the radius: arthroscopically assisted reduction compared with open reduction and internal fixation. J Bone Joint Surg 1999; 81(8):1093–1110.
8. Geissler WB, Freeland AE. Arthroscopically assisted reduction of intraarticular distal radius fractures. CORR 1996; 327:125–134.
9. Auge WK, Velazquez PA. The application of indirect reduction techniques in the distal radius: the role of adjuvant arthroscopy. Arthroscopy 2000; 16(8):830–835.
10. Buchko GM, Johnson DH. Arthroscopy assisted operative management of tibial plateau fractures. CORR 1996; 332:29–36.
11. Duwelius PJ, Rangitsch MR, Colville MR, et al. Treatment of tibial plateau fractures with limited internal fixation. CORR 1997; 339:47–57.
12. Carro LP, Nunez MP, Llata JI. Arthroscopic-assisted reduction and percutaneous external fixation of a displaced intraarticular glenoid fracture. Arthroscopy 1999; 15(2):211–214.
13. Sidor ML, Zuckerman JD, Lyon T, et al. The Neer Classification system for proximal humerus fractures. J Bone Joint Surg 1993; 75A:1745–1750.
14. Siebenrock KA, Gerber C. The reproducibility of classification of fractures of the proximal end of the humerus. J Bone Joint Surg 1993; 75A:1751–1755.
15. Park TS, et al. A new suggestion for the treatment of minimally displaced fractures of the greater tuberosity of the proximal humerus. Bull Hosp Joint Dis, 1997; 56(3):171–176.
16. Chen CY, Chao EK, Tu YK, et al. Closed management and percutaneous fixation of unstable proximal humerus fractures. J Trauma 1998; 45(6):1039–1045.
17. Jaberg H, Warner JJ, Jakob RP. Percutaneous stabilization of unstable fractures of the humerus. J Bone Joint Surg 1992; 74(4):508–515.

9

Ununited Fractures of the Clavicle and Proximal Humerus: Plate Fixation and Autogenous Bone Graft

DAVID RING and JESSE B. JUPITER

Harvard Medical School and Massachusetts General Hospital, Boston, Massachusetts, U.S.A.

I INTRODUCTION

Fractures of the clavicle and proximal humerus usually heal readily with little more than symptomatic treatment. Failure to heal often reflects substantial malalignment, soft tissue interposition, high-energy fractures with greater soft tissue injury, or excessive early motion (1,2). Operations to gain healing must enhance both the biological and mechanical aspects of fracture healing (3–5). The biological aspects of healing are addressed by limiting devascularization of fracture fragments during exposure, by debriding interposed tissue, by stimulating bleeding, by debriding and drilling the sclerotic fracture surfaces, and by adding autogenous bone graft. The mechanical aspects are addressed by applying adequate plate and screws.

II CLAVICLE

A Preoperative Planning

Radiographs will help determine if the nonunion is hypertrophic or atrophic. Hypertrophic nonunions will heal when stable fixation is applied. If a hypertrophic nonunion is associated with brachial plexus compression, the fracture site may need to be mobilized and the clavicle realigned to diminish encroachment of the callus on the thoracic outlet. If a hypertrophic nonunion follows an oblique fracture and is associated with shortening of the clavicle and dysfunction of the shoulder girdle, the surgeon might consider lengthening the clavicle by mobilizing the fracture site while maintaining apposition of the fragments through the oblique fracture (6). Shortening can be assessed by direct measurement of both clavicles on an anteroposterior chest radiograph or a radiograph including both shoulders with care taken to ensure that the shoulders are held in a comparable position and there is no rotation of the trunk (7,8).

An atrophic fracture (Fig. 1A) will require autogenous bone graft in addition to stable fixation. If the clavicle is shortened or there is a bony defect (as there often is in the setting of a synovial nonunion), it is advantageous to use a structural (tricortical) bone graft from the iliac crest (3). The size of the graft is estimated based upon preoperative measurements comparing the involved and uninvolved clavicle. This is best done on a radiograph without rotation that shows both clavicles.

B Operative Approaches

Operations suggested for the treatment of ununited fractures of the clavicle have included intramedullary fixation performed through an open exposure of the fracture site using an incision perpendicular to the clavicle (9), lengthening and plate fixation of an ununited oblique fracture (6), and wave plate fixation (intended to limit callus formation on the undersurface of the clavicle that might encroach on the thoracic outlet) (4). Our preferred approach is to debride, realign, bone graft, and plate the fracture through an incision in line with the clavicle. Surgeons have suggested applying the plate anteriorly or superiorly. We have used both, but usually apply the plate superiorly to avoid elevating attached muscles.

C Our Personal Approach

A slight beach chair position is used with the opposite iliac crest prepared (Fig. 1B). Exposure of the clavicle is performed through a straight incision in line with the clavicle and slightly inferior to it. Infiltration of the skin with a dilute epinephrine solution can help limit bleeding from the well-perfused skin of the shoulder girdle (Fig. 1C). Once the skin has been incised, dissection of the platysma and subcutaneous tissues is performed bluntly and under loupe magnification in order to identify and protect the supraclavicular nerves (Fig. 1D). A superior flap containing the skin, platysma, and the supraclavicular nerves is then elevated off of the clavicle. This provides sufficient exposure for application of a plate without elevating any muscles.

The fracture site is identified. If it is hypertrophic and there is no need to realign the fracture, a plate is applied without disturbing the fracture site. If the fracture is atrophic, the fracture site is opened and debrided of fibrous tissue and synovial membrane. The sclerotic fracture ends are then opened using a drill and the fracture edges debrided with a rongeur and curettes or a power burr to stimulate bleeding (Fig. 1E).

If realignment is needed, a small skeletal distractor is applied across the fracture site and gradual distraction is applied (Fig. 1E). If possible, the Schantz screws for the distractor should be applied so that they will not hinder plate application. Adherent tissues at the fracture site are elevated and incised to a limited extent to facilitate realignment of the fracture.

If a bone defect is present, the use of a structural graft will provide additional immediate support and limit callus formation (Fig. 1F). Excessive callus can encroach on the thoracic outlet. A cancellous graft is used for atrophic nonunions without bony defects. A bone graft is not usually needed for hypertrophic nonunions.

A plate is selected that provides three or four screws in the proximal and distal fragments. The plate is contoured and applied (Fig. 1G, H) The platysma and skin are then sutured (Fig. 1I, J). A drain is rarely necessary.

D Pearls and Pitfalls

Surgeons have expressed substantial concern regarding the potential for unsightly hypertrophic scars after operative exposure of the clavicle. We have used an incision in line with the clavicle with few problems.

Injury to one of the supraclavicular nerves can cause more than an annoying patch of numbness over the anterior chest wall; the pain associated with a neuroma is often disabling and has been associated with chronic regional pain syndromes (causalgia). With careful protection of these nerve branches, we have encountered few problems.

Limiting dissection of the clavicle is important not only for preservation of blood supply, but also to avoid injuring underlying structures such as the subclavian vein, brachial plexus, or lung. It is our impression that the use of a skeletal distractor to facilitate realignment and the use of an oscillating drill to protect neurovascular structures have greatly improved the safety of this procedure (Fig. 1E).

The structural (corticocancellous) bone graft can be contoured to enhance initial stability and healing. A tricortical graft that is larger than needed is obtained from the iliac crest. The ends of the graft are then trimmed to create pegs of cancellous bone (Fig. 1F). Troughs are created in the ends of the fracture fragments to accept these cancellous pegs. The graft is inserted upside down (i.e., superior cortex placed inferiorly) so that a screw can be placed into the graft through the plate. Avoid using 3.5 mm reconstruction plates. Although they are more malleable than dynamic and limited contact dynamic plates (DCP, LCDP), the reconstruction plates will often fail prior to nonunion healing.

E Postoperative Rehabilitation

Radiographs are taken prior to leaving the operating room and then every 2–4 weeks until the fracture is healed. In addition to the standard anteroposterior radiograph, it is often useful to obtain a view with the arm abducted. The clavicle rotates as the arm is abducted, and this rotation may improve visualization of the fracture site as the plate is rotated to a more directly superior position.

Patients wear a sling for comfort but are allowed functional mobilization of the arm the morning after surgery. Abduction and forward flexion of the shoulder above 90° are limited until early healing is established (4–6 weeks). Most patients will have no trouble regaining motion with simple physician-guided exercises and normal daily use of the arm. Patients with difficulty regaining motion are taught a set of active-assisted shoulder exercises by physical or occupational therapists.

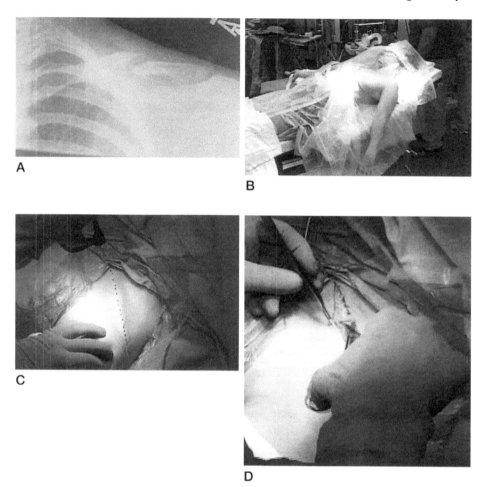

Figure 1 Plate and screw fixation for clavicle nonunion. (A) The pre-operative radiograph shows an atrophic nonunion with a bone defect. (B) The patient is placed in a beach chair position with the entire arm and chest wall and the contralateral iliac crest cleansed and included in the sterile field. (C) A straight incision, parallel to and just inferior to the clavicle is used. Infiltration of the skin with a dilute epinephrine mixture helps limit skin bleeding. (D) Blunt dissection of the subcutaneous tissue and platysma under loupe magnification helps to preserve the supraclavicular nerves. (E) A small distractor is used to help realign the clavicle. Fibrous and synovial tissues are debrided from the nonunion site. Sclerotic fracture surfaces are opened with a drill. (F) A corticocancellous bone graft taken from the iliac crest is contoured with pegs to interdigitate with the intramedullary canal of the fracture fragments. (G) A limited contact dynamic compression plate is contoured and applied to stabilize the clavicle. An attachment converts the drill to an oscillating drill. Oscillating drills are less likely to entangle soft tissue structures such as nerves, adding a measure of safety. (H) Autogenous cancellous bone graft is packed around the nonunion prior to closure of the platysma. (I) Closure of the platysma helps limit the prominence of the plate. (J) A subcuticular skin closure helps improve the appearance of the scar. (K) The graft is transfixed with a screw and stable, anatomical alignment of the clavicle.

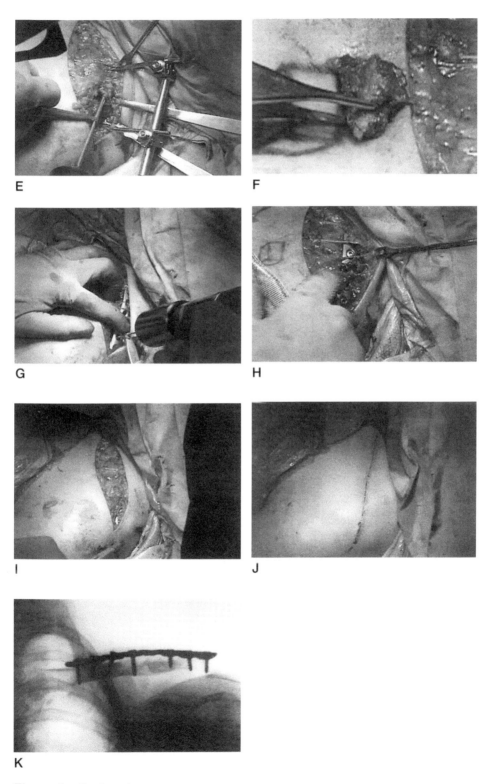

Figure 1 Continued.

III PROXIMAL HUMERUS

A Preoperative Planning

All atrophic nonunions—including those with a bony defect—require an autogenous cancellous bone graft. When there is a very large defect (>6 cm) and the soft tissue envelope is scarred and noncompliant, one might consider using a vascularized structural bone graft such as a free fibular graft. Restoration of length is not important in the humerus, but the dissection needed to bring the fracture fragments into apposition often devascularizes them. We prefer to preserve muscle and periosteal attachments to the bone and place autogenous bone graft into any defects.

Radiographs of the shoulder and humerus are used to determine optimal placement and length of the blade of the cannulated blade plate and the length of the side plate. Many patients with ununited fractures of the proximal humerus have poor bone quality, and the surgeon should be prepared for this. This may include having Schuhli washers (5,10) available and being familiar with their use. These washers fix the screw to the plate so that the hold in bone is not determined solely by engagement of the threads in the bone—instead, each screw becomes a fixed blade that would have to plow directly through the bone to loosen entirely. Some newer plate designs offer the ability to fix the screws to the plate through threads in the plate holes. Other methods for enhancing screw purchase include exchange of a 4.5 mm cortical screw to a 6.5 mm cancellous screw, the use of bone cement, and application of an allograft strut. Each of these bailout methods has drawbacks, and it is far better to anticipate poor bone quality and use screws that engage the plate.

With poor bone quality it is also important to use a very long plate. This not only enhances fixation, but also diminishes the risk that a fracture will occur at the distal limit of the plate (5).

Checchia and colleagues have classified nonunions of the proximal humerus into four groups (1): high two-part nonunions (Group 1), low two-part nonunions (Group 2), complex nonunions (Group 3), and lost fragments nonunions (Group 4). Group 3 and 4 nonunions are usually not amenable to operative fixation and are treated with hemiarthroplasty. The distinction between high and low nonunions is described in relation to the greater tuberosity, but may be difficult to apply reliably. Nonetheless, the concept of high and low nonunions is useful because high nonunions represent small articular fragments that are much more difficult to secure.

B Operative Approaches

Henry's extensile anterolateral exposure provides excellent exposure with little risk (11). Operative fixation of ununited fractures of the proximal humerus has been accomplished with a combination of intramedullary rods and sutures (12); with an allograft strut, plate, and screws (13); and with a standard plate or a blade plate and an autogenous bone graft (5,14) We prefer to use a blade plate and autogenous cancellous bone graft.

C Our Personal Approach

The skin is incised from the clavicle towards the insertion of the deltoid into its tuberosity on the humerus, passing just medial to the coracoid process (Figs. 2B, 3B). When a long plate is needed, the incision continues down the anterolateral aspect of the arm (Fig. 2B). The fascia over the deltoid and pectoralis major is exposed and the cephalic vein identified. This vein defines the deltopectoral interval. In most cases the vein is taken medially with the pectoralis major since the retraction of the deltoid required to expose the proximal humerus can be rough on the vein if it is taken laterally. The deltoid is elevated off of the humerus.

Distal dissection splits the brachialis with one third kept laterally and two thirds medial. The periosteum is preserved and the muscle is elevated minimally to accommodate a plate. When a long plate is used, it is worthwhile to find the radial nerve as it courses anteriorly between the brachialis and brachioradialis to be certain that it does not end up underneath the plate or get stretched excessively during the operation. The distal limit of the plate will be the coronoid and radial fossae.

Retraction of the deltoid can be facilitated by releasing a portion of the deltoid insertion. The insertion is very broad and the medial centimeter can safely be elevated. This also facilitates plate application. Again the elevation of this insertion should preserve periosteal attachments.

Adhesions in the subacromial bursa are mobilized when present, but release of the glenohumeral joint is not necessary.

The fracture site is identified and debrided of fibrous tissue. The fracture surfaces are debrided of sclerotic and devitalized bone (Fig. 2D). A drill is used to open the medullary canal of both fragments to encourage bleeding and the entrance of cells to participate in healing.

If there is malalignment of the fracture—particularly when there is overlapping in bayonet apposition—a skeletal distracter can be used to help realign the bone while limiting elevation of soft tissues (Fig. 2C).

We usually use a 4.5 mm cannulated blade plate or a 4.5 mm narrow LC-DCP bent into a blade plate. A 3.5 mm plate may be adequate in some instances. The position of the blade is carefully defined just below the tip of the greater tuberosity and the blade tract prepared, usually with drills. The plate is applied and screws applied; 6.5 mm cancellous screws are used in the head and 4.5 mm screws are placed in the diaphysis. After final wound irrigation, autogenous cancellous bone graft is placed in the fracture site and surrounding it. There is usually no need to suture the muscle intervals. The skin is closed over a suction drain, and a bulky dressing and a sling are applied.

D   Pearls and Pitfalls

Exposure of the radial nerve with very distal exposures may on occasion cause a temporary palsy. Patients should be aware of this. It is far better to undertake this risk than to risk more severe injury to the nerve by not knowing its exact location.

It is sometimes tempting to release part of the deltoid from the clavicle and acromion to improve proximal exposure. This should not be necessary and risks debilitating and very difficult to treat detachment of the deltoid. Partial elevation of the deltoid insertion and internal rotation of the proximal humerus fragment should be sufficient for blade insertion.

Use of a cannulated blade plate can greatly facilitate blade application. The wire for the blade is placed under image intensification and confirmed in multiple views. The length of the blade can be confirmed by measurement over the wire. The blade tract is drilled using a guide that fits over the wire and then a cannulated drill.

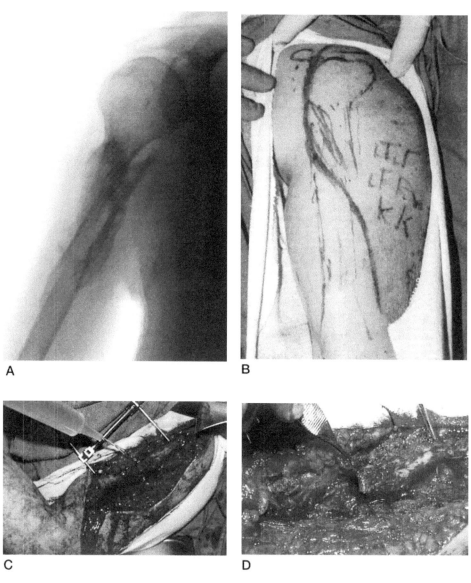

A   B

C   D

Figure 2 An unstable, synovial nonunion of the proximal humerus treated with plate and screw fixation and autogenous bone grafting. (A) Long oblique fractures of the proximal third are at greater risk of nonunion after functional bracing than transverse fractures and more distal fractures. (B) A deltopectoral skin incision is extended down the anterolateral aspect of the arm. (C) The brachialis is split, but muscle elevation is limited to that needed for plate application. A skeletal distractor is used for realignment. (D) Fibrous and synovial tissues were debrided and the sclerotic fracture ends opened with a rongeur and drill. (E) A tract for the blade of the blade plate is prepared using a drill. (F) The insertion of the deltoid is elevated slightly to improve plate position. (G) The final radiograph shows stable fixation with a blade plate. The use of 6.5 mm cancellous screws reflects poor bone quality. Now we would use a locking compression plate in which the screw locks into the plate. (H) The fracture healed and good flexion was restored.

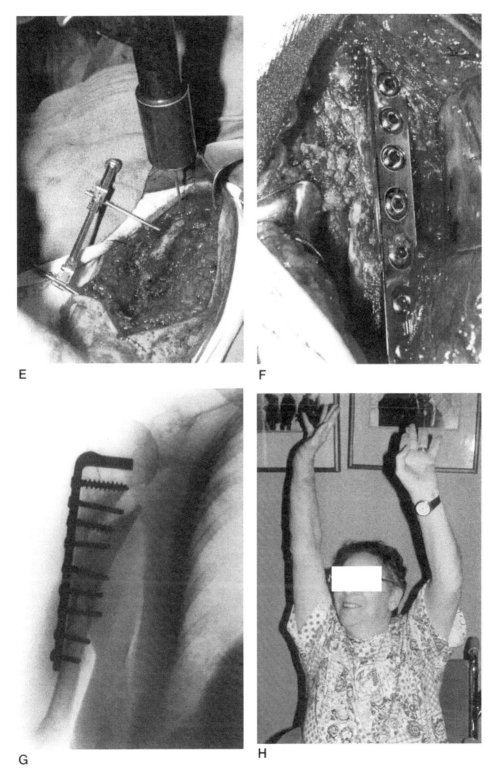

E

F

G

H

Figure 2 Continued.

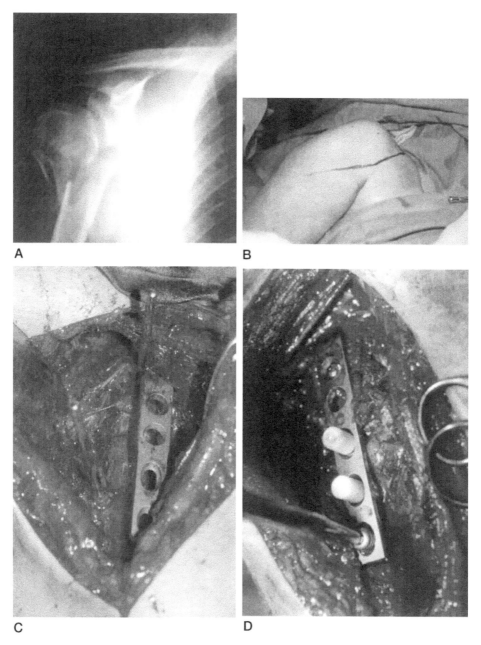

Figure 3 Osteoporosis can make plate and screw fixation of proximal humerus nonunions more difficult. (A) This anteroposterior radiograph shows an atrophic nonunion of the surgical neck of the humerus. (B) A deltopectoral approach extended into Henry's anterolateral exposure was used. (C) A skeletal distractor was used to facilitate realignment and the nonunion site debrided. Muscle and periosteal attachments were preserved. (D) Osteoporosis was anticipated and Schuhli nuts were used to convert the screws to fixed-angle devices. (E) The Schuhli nuts also bring the plate away from the bone, increasing the blood supply beneath the plate. (F) The final radiograph shows solid fixation. (G, H) Functional motion was obtained.

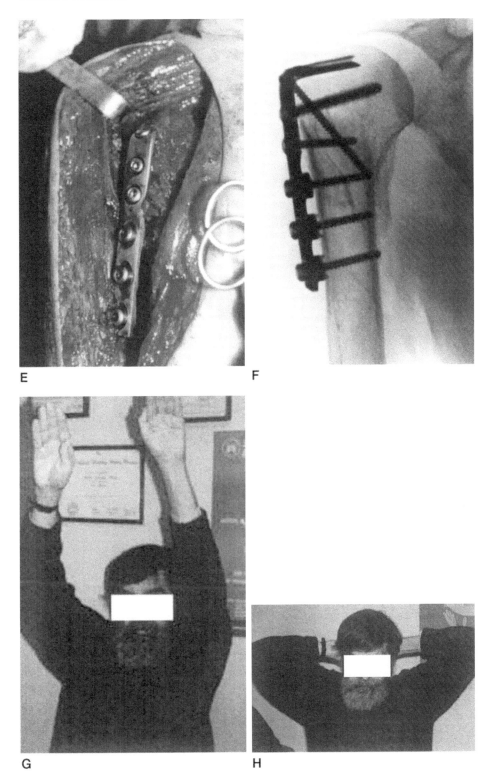

E

F

G

H

Figure 3 Continued.

Just as in the hip, the selection of the blade tract will determine how the plate lies on the bone and the alignment at the fracture site. Unlike in the hip, the blade does not need to have a tight fit. In fact, in osteoporotic bone it is risky to use force to impact the blade. The blade tract should therefore be prepared so that it is wide enough to slide the plate in and out fairly easily while still engaging the bone. It is also important to bevel the distal cortex so the bend of the plate does not impinge and crack the lateral cortex.

Poor bone quality should be anticipated so that screws that engage the plate can be used. Schuhli nuts can accomplish this (Fig. 3D). They are placed between the plate and bone and held temporarily with plastic screws. These are then sequentially exchanged for screws. A washer must be used with the screw to ensure that the threads engage (Fig. 3E). A newer plate design offers the possibility to thread screws directly into the plate. This type of plate can be bent into a blade plate.

For very proximal nonunions the strength of fixation is enhanced by placing a screw through the hole in the bend of the plate, directed obliquely and exiting the medial cortex of the distal fragment.

E Postoperative Rehabilitation

Patients are allowed immediate functional mobilization of the arm as comfort allows. Formal therapy is initiated when early healing is established, usually at 6 weeks. This focuses on active-assisted exercises including dowel-assist with the uninvolved arm.

IV CONCLUSIONS

The treatment of ununited fractures of the clavicle and proximal humerus consists of stable fixation of the fracture fragments without devascularizing them, stimulation of healing by debriding and drilling sclerotic fracture ends, and provision of autogenous bone graft. In the clavicle, realignment (including restoration of length) and protection of neurovascular structures including the supraclavicular nerves are important. In the proximal humerus, the surgeon must deal with poor quality bone and a relatively small proximal fragment. In both cases, rehabilitation focuses on active functional use of the limb initially. Once early healing is established, motion of the shoulder is usually predictably restored unless there is intrinsic pathology such as a rotator cuff problem or joint degeneration.

REFERENCES

1. Checchia SL, Doneux P, Miyanzaki AN, Spir IAZ, Bringel R, Ramos CH. Classification of nonunions of the proximal humerus. Int Orthop 2000; 24:217–220.
2. Hill JM, McGuire MH, Crosby LA. Closed treatment of displaced middle-third fractures of the clavicle gives poor results. J Bone Joint Surg 1997; 79:537–539.
3. Ring D, Jupiter JB. Ununited fractures of the clavicle: treatment with a sculptured corticocancellous iliac crest autogenous bone graft and plate fixation. Tech Hand Upper Extremity Surg. In press.
4. Ring D, Jupiter JB, Quintero J, Sanders R, Marti R. Atrophic ununited fractures of the humerus with bony defect: treatment with a bridging plate and autogenous cancellous bone graft. J Bone Joint Surg 2000; 832B:867.

5. Ring D, Perey B, Jupiter JB. The functional outcome of the operative treatment of ununited fractures of the humeral diaphysis in elderly patients. J Bone Joint Surg 1999; 81A:177–189.

6. Boyer MI, Axelrod TS. Atrophic nonunion of the clavicle: treatment by compression plate, lag-screw fixation and bone graft. J Bone Joint Surg 1997; 79B:301–303.

7. Eskola A, Vaininonpää S, Myllynen P, Pätiälä H, Rokkanen P. Outcome of clavicular fracture in 89 patients. Arch Orthop Trauma Surg 1986; 105:337–338.

8. Eskola A, Vaininonpää S, Myllynen P, Pätiälä H, Rokkanen P. Surgery for ununited clavicular fracture. Acta Orthop Scand 1986; 57:366–367.

9. Boehme D, Curtis RJ, DeHann JT, Kay SP, Young DC, Rockwood CA. Non-union of fractures of the mid-shaft of the clavicle. J Bone Joint Surg 1991; 73A:1219–1226.

10. Kolodziej P, Lee FS, Patel A, et al. Biomechanical evaluation of the Schuhli nut. Clin Orthop Rel Res 1998; 347:79–85.

11. Henry AK. Extensile Exposure. 2d ed. Edinburgh: Churchill Livingstone, 1973.

12. Duralde XA, Flatlow EL, Pollock RG, Nicholson GP, Self EB, Bigliani LU. Operative treatment of nonunions of the surgical neck of the humerus. J Should Elbow Surg 1996; 5:169–180.

13. Walch G, Badet R, Nove-Josserand L, Levigne C. Nonunions of the surgical neck of the humerus: surgical treatment with an intramedullary bone peg, internal fixation, and cancellous bone grafting. J Should Elbow Surg 1996; 5:161–168.

14. Jupiter JB, Mullaji AB. Blade plate fixation of proximal humeral non-unions. Injury 1994; 25:301–303.

10

Operative Treatment of Malunions of the Proximal Humerus

DAVID L. GLASER and MATTHEW L. RAMSEY

University of Pennsylvania and Hospital of the University of Pennsylvania, Philadelphia, Pennsylvania, U.S.A.

The management of proximal humeral malunions begins with understanding the etiological factors that led to the malunion and determining the current anatomy of the proximal humerus. This chapter is designed to assist orthopedic surgeons in the management of these complex problems, emphasizing the critical issues in a clinical and radiographic evaluation and making operative recommendations based on specific fracture malunion configurations.

I PREOPERATIVE PLANNING

A Clinical Evaluation

1 History

A careful history should determine the mechanism of injury and previous treatment with the goal of identifying contributing factors to the development of a malunion. Osteoporotic bone, inadequate fixation, premature or aggressive rehabilitation, and errors in diagnosis may have contributed to the malunion. Any pain or disability associated with the malunion must be assessed in terms of the patient's goals. A relatively painless malunion may not require surgical management, especially in a sedentary patient (1).

2 Physical Exam

Both active and passive arcs of motion must be evaluated. Loss of motion is a common problem complicating proximal humeral malunions (Fig. 1). Rotator cuff and deltoid function must be carefully evaluated to identify possible injury that may have occurred with the initial trauma or during prior failed surgeries. Assessment of

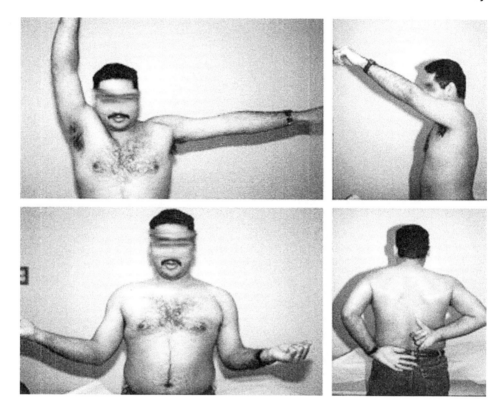

Figure 1   Limited range of motion following varus malunion of proximal humeral fracture. Loss of forward flexion, abduction, and external rotation is a common sequela of these types of fractures. This patient went on to have an osteotomy of the surgical neck with blade plate fixation. (Photographs courtesy of J. P. Iannotti, M.D., Ph.D.)

the degree of loss of both passive and active arcs of motion should be considered in terms of the patient's current disability and treatment goals. Good function can be achieved if the passive motion is maintained, the rotator cuff is intact, and the surface of the joint is congruent (2).

B   Implication of Malunion

A complete neurovascular examination of the involved upper extremity may identify permanent axillary nerve or brachial plexus injuries, especially if fracture fragments were initially displaced medial to the coracoid process (3). Axillary nerve injury is often associated with inferior subluxation of the proximal humerus (4). Electromyelographic examination can be helpful in determining the extent of injury and the prognosis for neurological recovery.

1   Radiographic Evaluation

Anteroposterior views in the plane of the scapula with the humerus in internal and external rotation, axillary, and scapular lateral views usually provide sufficient information to determine a treatment plan for most patients. Additional radio-

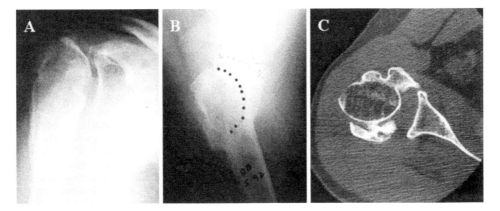

Figure 2 A 45-year-old businessman sustained a fall in India that was treated with nonoperative care. He only achieved 70° of elevation and 0° of external rotation and internal rotation to the buttock level. (A) Malunion of a four-part fracture is poorly defined on the anteroposterior view. (B) The axillary view improves the recognition of the displaced humeral head fragment (large dotted line), which is not congruent with the glenoid (small dotted line). (C) A CT scan best defines the marked displacement of the humeral head and the malunited tuberosities. (From Ref. 2.)

graphic views, such as the supraspinatus outlet view, may be helpful in the evaluation of greater tuberosity malunion. Computerized tomography is often useful when the plain radiographs are indeterminate or if detailed evaluation of articular congruity or fracture fragment displacement is needed (Fig. 2). Magnetic resonance imaging can demonstrate associated soft tissue problems of the deltoid, rotator cuff, biceps tendon, and glenoid labrum (Fig. 3).

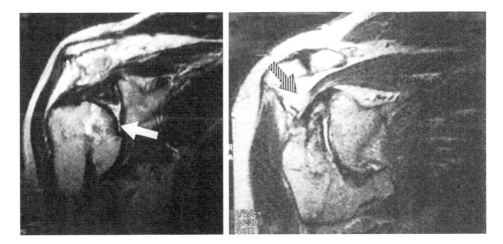

Figure 3 MRI of two different proximal humeral nonunions. MRI is useful in evaluating the humeral head for the presence of avascular necrosis or joint incongruity (solid white arrow). It is also useful to evaluate the rotator cuff for possible tears (striped arrow). (Photographs courtesy of J. P. Iannotti, M.D., Ph.D.)

II   OPERATIVE MANAGEMENT OF SPECIFIC PROXIMAL HUMERAL MALUNIONS

A   Two-Part Anatomical Neck Malunion

Isolated anatomical neck fractures are rare. An anatomical neck malunion can be treated by osteotomy and internal fixation, although risk of subsequent avascular necrosis would be a significant concern (Fig. 4). Hemiarthoplasty will usually achieve a more predictable result.

B   Two-Part Greater Tuberosity Malunion

Malunion of a greater tuberosity fracture is one of the most common proximal humeral malunions and can be extremely difficult to manage (5). The pattern of the malunion depends on the location of the fracture lines relative to the rotator cuff attachments to the tuberosity. Superior displacement of the greater tuberosity fragment occurs if there is unopposed pull of the supraspinatus on the fracture fragment. If the greater tuberosity fragment includes the infraspinatus attachment, then the fragment will retract posteriorly. Superior displacement is easily appreciated on an anteroposterior radiograph, while posterior displacement may be missed. The scapular lateral or axillary view is required to adequately demonstrate posterior displacement.

1   Surgical Indications

Chronically displaced, symptomatic greater tuberosity fractures should be managed surgically. A superiorly displaced greater tuberosity malunion may cause rotator cuff impingement and loss of forward elevation. As little as 5 mm of superior displacement in an active individual may result in symptoms of subacromial impingement. More sedentary patients with less than 10 mm displacement are observed expectantly. Posterior displacement of the tuberosity will result in weakness in external rotation and loss of external rotation as a result of tuberosity impingement on the glenoid. The motivation to consider surgical intervention is to improve pain and function.

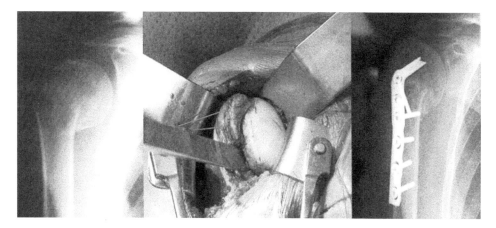

Figure 4   Varus malunion of a two-part anatomical neck fracture that was treated by open reduction, osteotomy, with blade plate fixation. (Photographs courtesy of J. P. Iannotti, M.D., Ph.D.)

2 Surgical Options

Several techniques are acceptable for treatment of these malunions. The superiorly displaced tuberosity may be managed with acromioplasty or osteotomy, mobilization, and anatomical reconstruction of the tuberosity. If the amount of displacement is small and the patient presents with symptoms that are predominantly impingement, acromioplasty is an acceptable treatment. Symptomatic posterior displacement requires osteotomy of the tuberosity, mobilization of the rotator cuff, and anatomical fixation of the tuberosity. Tuberosity mobilization to reestablish rotator cuff length and provide for a tension free repair can be extremely difficult. It requires circumferential release of the bursal and articular surfaces of the cuff. There are several methods to obtain tuberosity fixation. We prefer fixation with nonabsorbable sutures. However, internal fixation with screws and washers may be used in normal bone if the tuberosity fragment is large. The head of the screws should be placed lateral or distal to the greater tuberosity to avoid subacromial impingement. This method of fixation should be avoided in osteopenic bone. There is no place for a plate fixation in the management of a greater tuberosity malunion because of the space constraints of the subacromial area. Wire fixation does not seem to offer any distinct advantage over heavy nonabsorbable suture but does have the disadvantage of material failure and subsequent migration requiring removal.

3 Authors' Preferred Surgical Technique

If the degree of displacement is minimal and the patient's symptoms are primarily impingement, we prefer arthroscopic acromioplasty. This will not be discussed in detail in this chapter.

Displaced greater tuberosity malunions should be approached surgically in a method similar to an acute fracture. An incision parallel with the lateral edge of the acromion and centered 1 cm medial to the anterolateral corner of the acromion is recommended. The raphe between the anterior and middle deltoid is split for distance of 4 cm from the acromion and carried anteriorly by subperiosteally elevating the anterior deltoid off of the acromion. Subacromial scar tissue is excised when present. The greater tuberosity fragment is identified by digital palpation or direct inspection by opening the rotator interval. Once identified, the tuberosity fragment is mobilized by dissection of a fibrous malunion or by osteotomy of a bony malunion. Articular and bursal sided rotator cuff mobilization reestablishes cuff length, allowing anatomical fixation of the tuberosity. The ability to reestablish rotator cuff length can be extremely difficult if the degree of medial displacement is significant. In cases where it cannot be anatomically reduced, the greater tuberosity is mobilized laterally as far as possible and below the top of the humeral head.

Fragment fixation can be performed with suture, wire, or screws. Screw fixation is a reasonable fixation option when the bone quality is good and the fragment size is large enough to accommodate the screws without comminuting the fragment. For all other patients, we prefer suture fixation. (Fig. 5) The fragment is held in place using two to four heavy, nonabsorbable sutures, placed in a figure-eight configuration through the greater tuberosity. This provides horizontal fixation of the greater tuberosity to the humeral head/lesser tuberosity and vertical fixation to the humeral shaft. We prefer heavy nonabsorbable suture placed at the tendon-bone junction in order to avoid suture cutout of the tuberosity. Interosseous sutures with a

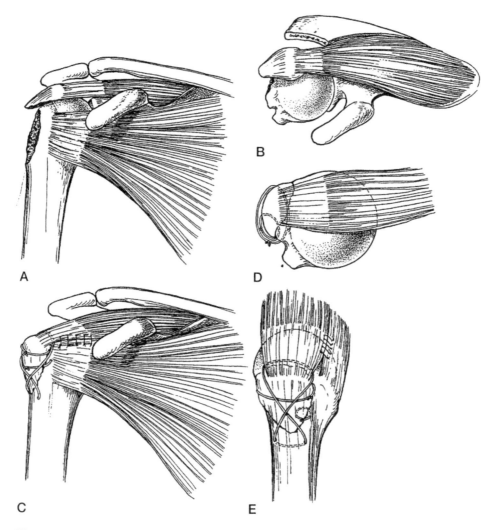

Figure 5 (A and B) Isolated greater tuberosity malunion with superoposterior displacement. (C–E) Reduction of the greater tuberosity and internal fixation using transosseous horizontal sutures and vertical figure-of-eight sutures. The horizontal sutures between the tuberosities are placed between the bone fragments, which helps to reduce the fragments, and in the rotator cuff tendon insertion sites, which provides the best tissue for maintaining the reduction during the postoperative evaluation. The vertical figure-of-eight suture also passes through the tendon insertion site and then passes through a drill hole 2 cm distal to the metaphyseal fracture line. The vertical suture prevents superior displacement. The rotator interval between the subscapularis and supraspinatus is repaired, significantly improving stability. (From Ref. 2.)

figure-eight configuration through the fracture site can aid in fragment reduction and prevent overlap.

4   Postoperative Management

Passive supine elevation and external rotation motion is begun the day of surgery, but internal rotation behind the back and extension is avoided for 6 weeks. Active motion is begun at 6 weeks, followed by resistance exercises.

C   Two-Part Lesser Tuberosity Malunion

Two-part lesser tuberosity fractures are rare but are often associated with posterior shoulder dislocations. Medial pull of the subscapularis will tend to retract the fragment medially. If the fragment is large and the rotator interval is torn at the time of injury, medial retraction can be considerable. The malunited fragment may act as an obstacle to internal rotation and may also involve the articular surface of the humeral head.

Orthogonal radiographs, especially the axillary view, are usually sufficient to diagnose the size of the fragment and degree of medial retraction. Computed tomography (CT) scans can assist in determining size and displacement of the fragment if standard radiographs do not provide the necessary information.

1   Authors' Preferred Surgical Technique

An extended deltopectoral approach is utilized. Internal fixation can be achieved utilizing heavy nonabsorbable sutures or screws. The choice of the method of fixation parallels that in greater tuberosity malunions. Care is taken to achieve anatomical reduction of associated articular fragments. Intraosseous fixation to the greater tuberosity passing deep to the bicipital groove can also be used. Small lesser tuberosity fragment can be excised and the subscapularis tendon repaired directly to the proximal humerus. A chronically retracted fragment may require release on both sides of the subscapularis tendon and mobilization of the rotator interval and inferior surface. The capsule can be safely released from the inner aspect of the joint near the glenoid margin. Inferior capsular release from the subscapularis requires identification and protection of the axillary nerve.

2   Postoperative Management

Passive supine elevation and external rotation motion is begun the day of surgery. Intraoperatively, the safe zone of external rotation is defined and not exceeded in the first 6 weeks postoperatively until tuberosity healing is begun. Internal rotation behind the back is avoided for 6 weeks. Active motion is begun at 6 weeks, followed by resistance exercises.

D   Surgical Neck Malunion

Surgical neck malunions occur from the unopposed pull of the pectoralis major and rotator cuff resulting in combined apex anterior angulation and varus deformity. Varus deformity places the greater tuberosity prominently in the subacromial space leading to impingement.

Diagnosis is readily made utilizing standard radiographs. However, if x-rays do not show all of the features of the malunion, a CT scan may be helpful.

1   Authors' Preferred Surgical Technique

If clinically indicated, osteotomy and internal plate fixation are performed at the malunion site. Osteotomy must be carefully planned to correct the multiplane deformity present. The requirement for internal fixation is the ability to achieve immediate, stable internal fixation that permits early range of motion. In patients with good bone quality, we prefer a blade plate. Other options for internal fixation include tension band techniques with or without intramedullary rods (Fig. 6). Open capsular release is usually necessary to restore satisfactory passive arcs of motion and is performed before osteotomy.

An extended deltopectoral approach is utilized. The axillary nerve is identified anteriorly and followed posteriorly to the quadrilateral space. This amount of dissection is required to protect the nerve during osteotomy. A biplane osteotomy to correct the varus and apex anterior angulation is undertaken. Bone from the osteotomy can be used for the graft or some bone graft substitute. For patients with intra-articular fracture or posttraumatic arthritis, hemiarthroplasty is recommended.

E   Three- and Four-Part Malunions

Three- and four-part malunions are the result of complex bony and soft tissue abnormalities (Fig. 7). In order to achieve a satisfactory result in the treatment of malunited three- and four-part fractures, all bony and soft tissue abnormalities must be identified and addressed at the time of surgery. Bony abnormalities can affect the

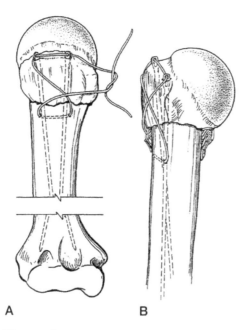

A   B

Figure 6   Technique of internal fixation of a neck malunion. The humeral head is impacted to improve fracture stability. In some cases, multiple suture fixation after impaction of the shaft into an osteoporotic head can be used. (Photographs courtesy of J. P. Iannotti, M.D., Ph.D.)

tuberosities, shaft, or articular segment. Soft tissue abnormalities include capsular contracture, scarring or defects of the rotator cuff, or neurovascular deficits.

Treatment of three- and four-part malunions can include osteotomy and realignment of the malunited segments around the articular segment with internal fixation or prosthetic replacement (Fig. 8). In selected three-part injuries, osteotomy of the fracture fragments followed by internal fixation may be attempted if there is good bone quality, no humeral head avascular necrosis, or joint incongruity. If the malunion involves several component parts, the difficulty of osteotomy and realignment may make prosthetic replacement a more predictable option.

Surgeons should inform patients preoperatively of the postoperative prognosis, and both the surgeon and the patient should have limited goals (6–8). Tuberosity management remains controversial (9,10). However, it begins with determination of tuberosity position. CT scan is often helpful.

1 Authors' Preferred Surgical Technique

The goal of treating three- and four-part proximal humerus malunions is to reestablish the normal anatomical relationships of the tuberosity, shaft, and head fragments. The integrity of the glenoid articular surface determines whether humeral hemiarthroplasty or total shoulder arthroplasty is performed.

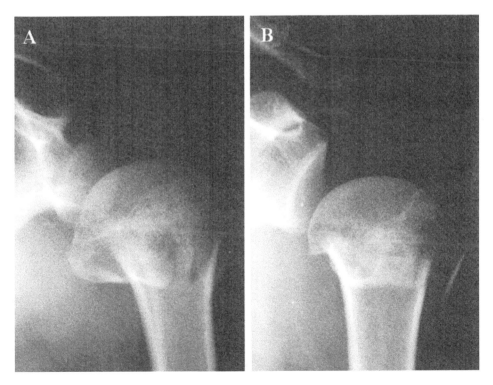

Figure 7 Internal and external rotation views of a four-part valgus impacted malunion showing current positions of the tuberosities and head fragments. This fracture was treated with a hemiarthroplasty. (Photographs courtesy of J. P. Iannotti, M.D., Ph.D.)

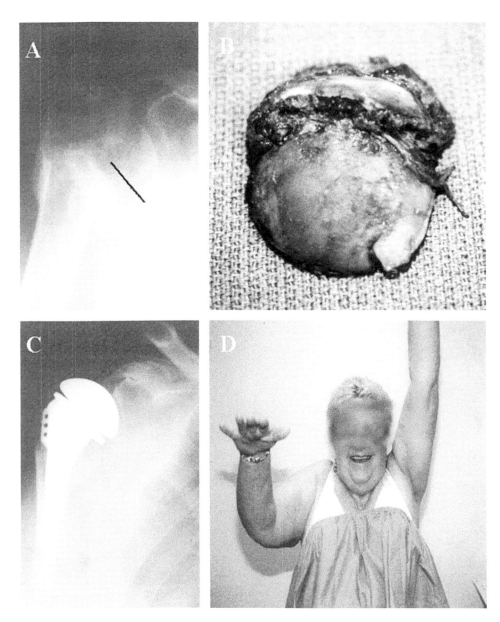

Figure 8 Humeral head-splitting, three-part malunion. Conservative management (A) of this fracture led to articular incongruity (B), persistent pain, and loss of function. A hemiarthroplasty (C) was able to restore proper alignment and tuberosity height without the need for a tuberosity osteotomy. The black line (A) demonstrates the level of neck cut used to ensure that both the lesser and greater tuberosities remain below the collar of the prosthesis. At follow-up, the patient had no pain, but active elevation was limited because of weakness resulting from an axillary nerve neurapraxia (D). (Adapted from Ref. 2.)

An extensive deltopectoral approach with lysis of any subacromial and subdeltoid scarring is used. Capsular contracture always exists, and an extensive capsular release is required. Rotator cuff and capsule mobilization can be enhanced by surgical release of the capsule near the glenoid rim. The rotator cuff should be carefully inspected for tears, and these should be repaired.

Tuberosity position must be assessed intraoperatively. Greater tuberosity malunion often blocks external rotation or forward elevation. Lesser tuberosity malunion may permit excessive posterior subluxation or block internal rotation because of coracoid process impingement. While restoration of the normal anatomical relationships is directly related to overall function, reconstructing these relationships is no longer done at all costs. With improvement of prosthesis design, adapting the prosthesis to the distorted anatomy will most likely play a more significant role in the management of these malunions. A modular shoulder arthroplasty system, with a number of neck and head component sizes, options, angles, and offsets, will often allow satisfactory prosthetic placement, avoiding the need for tuberosity osteotomy. Large degrees of tuberosity displacement still require osteotomy. The bicipital groove is a helpful landmark for tuberosity osteotomy. The osteotomy should produce a tuberosity fragment long enough to ensure contact with the humeral shaft on repositioning and large enough so that adequate rotator cuff is attached. The attached rotator cuff may need to be mobilized to achieve needed length.

Tuberosity fixation is achieved by using several heavy, nonabsorbable sutures. Two sutures are passed through the middle portion of the tuberosities and the anterior or lateral flange of the prosthesis. Two more sutures are passed through both tuberosities, one each at the superior and inferior ends. An anteroposteriorly directed hole is drilled through the lateral aspect of the proximal humeral shaft. Two sutures are passed through this hole and, in figure-eight fashion, passed through the superior aspect of the tuberosities at the cuff insertion. These two sutures assist in bringing the tuberosities inferior to ensure contact of the tuberosities and the humeral shaft. Local bone graft is usually available from the discarded head fragment and is used to assist tuberosity healing. Impingement can be avoided by making certain that the tuberosities are below the superior level of the humeral head.

REFERENCES

1. Siegel JA, Dines DM. Proximal humerus malunions. Orthop Clin North Am 2000; 31:35–50.
2. Iannotti JP, Sidor ML. Malunions of the proximal humerus. In: Warner JJP, Iannotti JP, Gerber C, eds. Complex and Revision Problems in Shoulder Surgery. Philadelphia: Lippincott-Raven Publishers, 1997:245–264.
3. McLaughlin JA, Light R, Lustrin I. Axillary artery injury as a complication of proximal humerus fractures. J Shoulder Elbow Surg 1998; 7:292–294.
4. Perlmutter GS. Axillary nerve injury. Clin Orthop Related Res 1999; 368:28–36.
5. Beredjiklian PK, Iannotti JP, Norris TR, Williams GR. Operative treatment of malunion of a fracture of the proximal aspect of the humerus. J Bone Joint Surg Am 1998; 80:1484–1497.
6. Gobel F, Wuthe T, Reichel H. [Results of shoulder hemiarthroplasty in patients with acute and old fractures of the proximal humerus]. Z Orthop Grenzgeb 1999; 137:25–30.

7. Beredjiklian PK, Iannotti JP. Treatment of proximal humerus fracture malunion with prosthetic arthroplasty. Instr Course Lect 1998; 47:135–140.

8. Norris TR, Green A, McGuigan FX. Late prosthetic shoulder arthroplasty for displaced proximal humerus fractures. J Shoulder Elbow Surg 1995; 4:271–280.

9. Boileau P, Trojani C, Walch G, Krishnan SG, Romeo A, Sinnerton R. Shoulder arthroplasty for the treatment of the sequelae of fractures of the proximal humerus. J Shoulder Elbow Surg 2001; 10:299–308.

10. Frankle MA, Greenwald DP, Markee BA, Ondrovic LE, Lee WE, 3rd. Biomechanical effects of malposition of tuberosity fragments on the humeral prosthetic reconstruction for four-part proximal humerus fractures. J Shoulder Elbow Surg 2001; 10:321–326.

11

Treatment of Locked Anterior and Posterior Dislocations of the Shoulder

SERGIO L. CHECCHIA

Santa Casa Hospitals and School of Medicine, São Paulo, Brazil

I INTRODUCTION

Although traumatic dislocations of the shoulder, either anterior or posterior, are not rare, the diagnosis is frequently missed. It is not uncommon to find patients whose diagnosis has not been made for many months and whose treatment may therefore not have been appropriate. Patients with anterior dislocations of the shoulder tend to seek medical attention earlier, presenting with typical signs and symptoms. The clinical scenario with posterior dislocations, however, is altogether different. Patients' presenting symptoms are often less clear-cut, and an inexperienced examiner may miss the diagnosis. It is surprising, however, that posterior dislocations are missed so frequently considering that Cooper (1), in 1839, carefully warned about this condition. He stated: "It's an accident that cannot be mistaken, as there is a protuberance formed by the bone upon the scapula, which immediately strikes the eye."

II LOCKED ANTERIOR FRACTURE-DISLOCATION OF THE SHOULDER

A Acute Cases: Preoperative Planning

Anterior fracture-dislocations of the shoulder in older patients who may have weak tendons of the rotator cuff and osteopenia are associated with increased complications. The most frequent complication is a rotator cuff tear, or even an extension of a previous lesion. The tendons that are commonly involved are the supraspinatus and infraspinatus tendons. Therefore, every patient over 40 years of age that presents with pain after having a reduction of an anterior shoulder dislocation should be suspected of having an associated rotator cuff tear.

Neurological lesions may also occur, but are less common than rotator cuff tears. The axillary nerve is most frequently affected. In most cases, it presents only as a neurapraxia, therefore, complete recovery is expected in 3 or 4 months (2). It is important to be aware of these concurrent injuries, especially when the dislocation is associated with severe rotator cuff tears, since the recovery may be slower due to the neurological lesion. In these cases, magnetic resonance imaging (MRI) should always be performed to adequately evaluate the extension of the tear and the tendons involved (Fig. 1). Rupture of the subscapularis tendon and medial dislocation of the biceps tendon may also occur, which may cause severe pain and functional impairment (Fig. 2).

Patients with acute rotator cuff tears and inability to actively elevate the arm should be treated operatively as early as possible. Nonoperative treatment of the neurological lesion is usually appropriate since spontaneous neurological recovery is expected to occur. However, this will depend on the patient's age and clinical status.

The pathology should dictate the approach: if the primary pathology involves the anterior structures (subscapularis, labrum), then a deltopectoral approach is

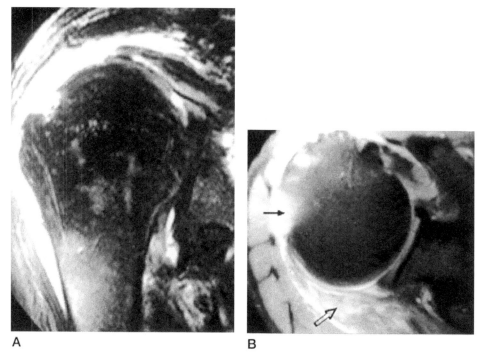

A   B

Figure 1   MRI image of a 54-year-old male with a massive rotator cuff tear following a traumatic locked anterior dislocation. (A) Large supraspinatus tendon tear and edema in the joint. (B) The bold arrow indicates a Hill-Sachs lesion and the outlined arrow shows the associated infraspinatus tendon involvement.

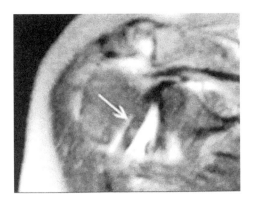

Figure 2 MRI image of a 63-year-old female showing dislocation of the biceps tendon (white arrow) and a subscapularis tendon tear following traumatic locked anterior dislocation.

favored. The skin incision can be extended into an anterosuperior incision (off the lateral aspect of the deltoid) if necessary, and the deltoid can be incised off of the anterior aspect of the acromion. Anterior instability can occur in these patients, and if the Bankart lesion is large, we recommend repairing it. On the other hand, if the labral lesion is small and there is a large posterior rotator cuff tear, then a primary rotator cuff repair will usually suffice.

B Chronic Cases

Despite the evident deformity and functional impairment caused by anterior shoulder dislocations, one may sometimes encounter a neglected chronic case. These cases are very difficult to manage, due to the lesion itself and also often due to patient noncompliance.

1 Imaging

Radiographic examination will usually confirm the diagnosis when the trauma series is obtained. This includes an AP view in the plane of the scapula, a lateral view in the plane of the scapula, and an axillary view. Imaging should enable evaluation of the size of the Hill-Sachs lesion. Computed tomography (CT) scans and MRIs can also aid in the diagnosis, but may be confusing at times because images of several different levels of the joint are obtained. In the author's opinion, a complete trauma series including an axillary view is sufficient, but in some cases a CT scan may help in identifying associated lesions such as fractures or erosions of the anterior border of the glenoid (Fig. 3A–C). An MRI may also be used to evaluate the degree of muscular atrophy and/or associated rotator cuff lesions.

2 Classification

The duration of time between the injury and the diagnosis is critical in order to adequately treat these injuries. Hawkins divided chronic dislocations into three groups, and we feel that this classification is quite useful (3). Group I injuries occurred within the previous 6 months, Group II injuries 6–12 months previously,

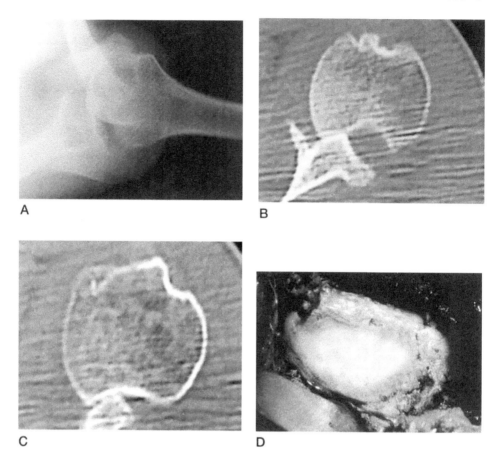

Figure 3 Image of 43-year-old male with locked anterior dislocation: (A) axillary x-ray revealing a large Hill-Sachs lesion and erosion of the anterior border of the glenoid; (B and C) CT scan in different levels of this shoulder showing different sizes of Hill-Sachs lesions and of erosion of the anterior border of the glenoid; (D) operative view demonstrating large erosion of the anterior border of the glenoid; (E) correction with iliac crest bone grafting; (F) final x-ray imaging the screws and the anchors used to suture the capsule to the border of the glenoid.

and Group III injuries greater than 12 months before the time of diagnosis. At 6 months there may still be preservation of the joint cartilage; after this period, however, degeneration of the articular cartilage begins to occur; and after 12 months irreversible damage to the glenoid cartilage occurs (Table 1).

3 Operative Approaches

Treatment of these difficult lesions depends on several factors, including delay in diagnosis, severity of associated lesions, and the patient's overall status and expectations.

Table 1 Hawkins' Classification for Chronic Locked Anterior Fracture-Dislocation of the Shoulder (LADS)

Group	Time[a]	Proposed treatment
I	<6 months	Open reduction and Bankart repair
II	>6 months but <12 months	Hemiarthroplasty
III	>12 months	Total shoulder

[a] Time between accident and treatment.

Group I: Dislocations 3 Weeks–6 Months. In patients who present greater than 3 weeks from the injury, the best treatment is open reduction. This minimizes the possibility of incurring diaphyseal fractures, humeral head impaction fractures, or even iatrogenic neurovascular lesions (Fig. 4). The patient is placed in the beach chair position, and the extremity is draped free. The operation should be carried out carefully with extensive soft tissue release. Release of the entire joint and coracohumeral ligament is often mandatory in these cases. Wide exposure is necessary for these procedures; thus, we perform a tenotomy of the conjoined tendon to easily identify and protect the axillary and musculocutaneous nerves, besides

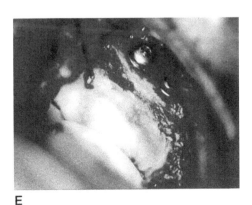
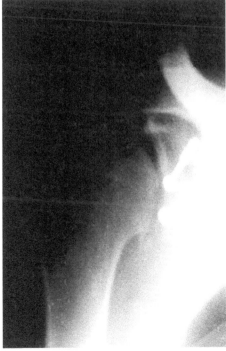

E   F

Figure 3 Continued.

palpating the brachial plexus. We feel that conjoined tendon release aids tremendously in reduction of the humeral head and decreases the possible neurovascular complications that can occur due to the altered anatomy.

Once the shoulder is reduced, stability is achieved by repairing the labral lesion (Bankart lesion). One must carefully examine the anterior border of the glenoid since fracture and erosion often occur and may require bone graft supplementation (Fig. 3). Following this repair, a capsular shift (if necessary) is carried out in approximately 20–30° of external rotation. When severe capsular damage has occurred, the subscapularis tendon can be incorporated with the Bankart lesion suture. This will most likely limit external rotation; however, this is more preferable than residual subluxation. Gerber (4) has reported good results using homologous bone graft fixed with screws to treat large Hill-Sachs lesions. We have avoided this technique, however, due to concern about graft necrosis and the potential of loose hardware in the joint.

Group II: Delay in Diagnosis of 6–12 Months. When dislocations are over 6 months old, there will inevitably be degeneration of the cartilage of the humeral head and/or weakness of the subchondral bone (Fig. 5). Hemiarthroplasty is the appropriate choice in these cases. Soft tissue balancing is quite challenging, however, due to the contraction of the capsule and soft tissue constraints. For example, a posterior capsular release is often necessary following osteotomy of the humeral neck for placement of the prosthesis. After the trial component is placed, the shoulder is kept in forced internal rotation for a few minutes in order to stretch the posterior structures, which will in turn increase stability.

It is of utmost importance to accurately determine the exact version of the prosthesis. The greatest challenge lies in determining the proper retroversion in which the prosthesis should be placed. The perception is that one should increase the retroversion due to the fixed anterior dislocation. However, excessive retroversion,

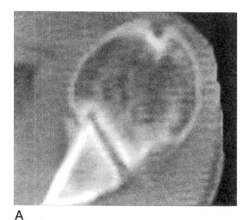 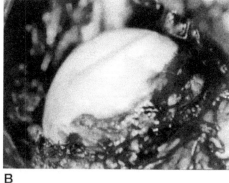

A   B

Figure 4   Image of 42-year-old female with a 2-month-old locked anterior dislocation who underwent closed reduction. (A) CT scan image showing flattening of the head after reduction and (B) operative view of the humeral head flattening.

especially in conjunction with a posterior capsular release, may lead to posterior dislocation of the prosthesis. Therefore, we recommend a humeral head resection in 30° of retroversion, and then stability should be tested with the trial component. If necessary, this retroversion may gradually be increased. When the prosthesis has a modular eccentric head, it may be placed with a more posterior offset (Fig. 6). Achieving balance between stability and mobility is the greatest challenge facing the surgeon. In most cases, patients are kept immobilized in internal rotation for a few weeks after surgery. However, prolonged immobilization may lead to decreased postoperative range of motion. Deliz and Flatow (5) reported seven excellent, two good, and one satisfactory result with this technique.

Group III: Dislocations 12 Months Old.   When dislocations are greater than 12 months old, a total shoulder replacement is likely to be required, since irreversible damage to the glenoid cartilage is expected. Occasionally erosions of the glenoid border may impede arthroplasty. Achieving a stable and functional total shoulder replacement in these patients is extremely difficult due to the duration of the dislocation and the resultant soft tissue contractures. The author's experience in these cases has been disappointing (6). Four patients with shoulder dislocations greater than 12 months were treated surgically—two with fair results and the other 2 with poor results, according to the UCLA shoulder rating score.

Considering the poor outcome of these patients, one may consider alternative treatments, such as arthrodesis or even humeral head resection. However, sometimes these patients present with little or no pain and satisfactory to reasonable function (Fig. 7). In such cases the best management is "skillful neglect treatment" (5).

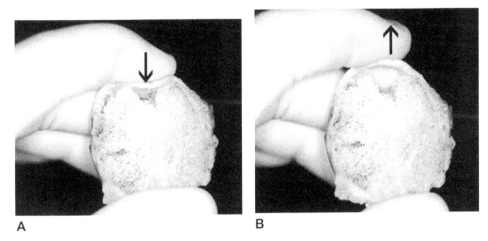

A   B

Figure 5   Surgical specimen of a 6-month-old locked anterior dislocation. (A) Note the weakness of the subchondral bone and how the cartilage deforms when pressed; (B) recovery of the cartilage's original shape when pressure is removed; this is the so-called ping-pong ball head.

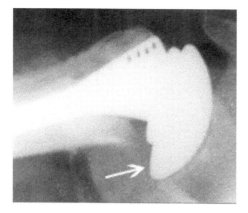

Figure 6 X-ray of a locked anterior dislocation case treated with an eccentric head prosthesis placed with a more posterior offset.

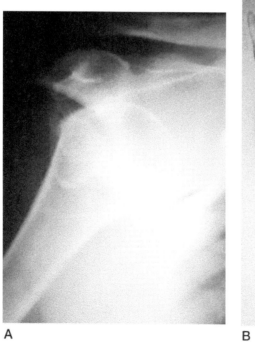

A

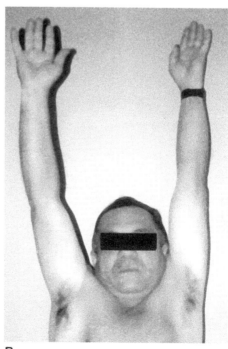

B

Figure 7 Patient with a 4-year-old neglected locked anterior dislocation presenting with minimal complaints of pain: (A) x-ray; (B) function.

4 Postoperative Rehabilitation

Radiographs are obtained in all cases at 1, 3, and 6 weeks postoperatively for Group I patients. Group II and Group III patients, however, require yearly radiographs to check the status of the prosthesis and identify any signs of early failure (lysis, change of position, glenoid wear).

Group I patients will have their therapy directed based on the operative findings and procedure performed. If a standard Bankart procedure is all that is necessary to achieve stability, passive and active-assisted forward elevation and external rotation can commence at approximately 2 weeks postoperatively. The limits are determined on the intraoperative findings, but in general we allow forward elevation to ~ 90–$130°$ and forward elevation to $30°$ in the first 2–4 weeks. The limits are increased to 130–$170°$ and 30–$60°$, respectively, from weeks 4–6. Active elevation and external rotation are delayed until 6 weeks so that the subscapularis and the labral repair can adequately heal. Stregthening exercises are then begun and continued for 3–6 months postoperatively.

Group II and Group III patients require much slower rehabilitation due to the concerns outlined above. These patients may require the use of an orthosis (such as a gunslinger) to keep the shoulder reduced while the soft tissues heal following the extensive releases necessary to achieve balance and stability. If stability is not an issue, then carefully supervised passive and active-assisted forward elevation and external rotation can begin by 2–4 weeks following the procedure. Active exercises are withheld for at least 6–8 weeks in these patients and are usually not initiated until weeks 10–12 to allow adequate healing.

III LOCKED POSTERIOR FRACTURE-DISLOCATION OF THE SHOULDER

A Preoperative Planning

In this section we will discuss acute and chronic posterior dislocations of the shoulder together. In both types of dislocation, factors other than the time of history alone are important for proper management. In these cases the presence of associated bone lesions is also important. In some situations the same surgical procedure can be used to treat acute or chronic posterior dislocations.

B Imaging

Radiographic classification and treatment are based on the presence of lesions in the anteromedial aspect of the humeral head, the so-called McLaughlin lesion, as well as the time from injury to diagnosis. Therefore, the trauma radiographic series is fundamental for the diagnosis and management of these lesions. An axillary view is important for the diagnosis of the original lesion and of associated lesions as well. It enables classification according to the size of the humeral head fracture and helps to determine adequate treatment (Fig. 8).

C Classification

In 1970 Neer published a classic paper on fractures of the proximal humerus and proposed a classification for locked posterior fracture-dislocation of the shoulder (LPDS) based on the size of the McLaughlin lesion (7). In 1985 Hawkins added the

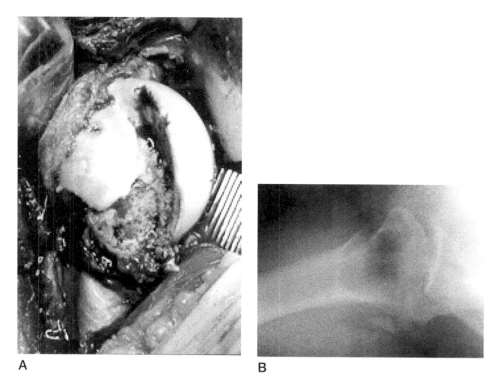

A   B

Figure 8   McLaughlin lesion: (A) surgical view; (B) axillary view. Measurement of the size of the lesion is easier and more accurate using axial images than using intraoperative measurements.

time factor to Neer's classification, since the duration from injury to diagnosis is extremely important to determine the appropriate type of treatment (3). We have proposed a classification (see Table 2) based on the pathology and the duration of time from the accident to the treatment in order to classify locked posterior dislocation in a more objective and broad manner (8).

D   Operative Management

1   Group I: Closed Reduction and Immobilization in External Rotation

When less than 20% of the humeral head is involved and the lesion is less than 4 weeks old, patients are treated with closed reduction under anesthesia and immobilization in external rotation of approximately 30°. It is impossible to perform a closed reduction, however, in cases where the biceps tendon is interposed (9). Immobilization should be maintained for 6 weeks (10). In our experience, patients treated according to this protocol had excellent results with little loss of motion, even after immobilization of 6 weeks. Dubousset (11) also had all excellent outcomes using this treatment modality in 12 shoulders at long follow-up.

Table 2 Classification for Locked Posterior Fracture-Dislocation of the Shoulder (LPDS)

Group		Lesion	Time[a]	Proposed treatment
I		<20%	Acute	Closed reduction and immobilization in ER for 6 weeks
II		2-part tuberosity fracture		
		3-part fracture Anatomical neck fracture[b]	Acute	ORIF
III		>20% but <50%	Acute or chronic <6 months	McLaughlin's procedure or Neer's modification
		>50%		
	A	4-part fracture Anatomical neck fracture[b]	Acute or chronic <6 months	
IV				Hemiarthroplasty
	B	Abnormal humeral head cartilage	Chronic <12 months	
V		Osteoarthritis	Chronic <2 years	Total shoulder
VI		Very severe osteoarthritis	Chronic >2 years	Arthrodesis Resection arthroplasty Rehabilitation

[a] Time between accident and treatment.
[b] Anatomical neck fractures can be treated: for young patients, ORIF (anatomical reduction is mandatory); for older patients, hemiarthroplasty.

2 Group II: Open Reduction and Internal Fixation

Some acute cases, such as three- or four part fracture-dislocations or fractures of the anatomical neck, require immediate surgical treatment. Neer (7) reported on four three-part locked posterior dislocations treated with open reduction and internal fixation (ORIF) and had an excellent result in two cases, a satisfactory result in one case, and one patient who developed nonunion.

We find that young patients with locked posterior dislocations associated with fracture of the anatomical neck can be treated with ORIF through a careful anterior approach with minimal soft tissue damage and fixation of the humeral head with two lag screws. A deltopectoral approach is used, and the rotator interval is opened followed by an incision, no greater than 1–1.5 cm, of the subscapularis tendon to enable delicate reduction of the fracture (Fig. 9).

Caution must be taken with a specific locked posterior dislocation where the McLaughlin lesion is associated with a complete non-displaced fracture of the anatomical neck. It is nearly impossible to safely reduce the dislocation without displacing the anatomical neck making the prognosis much worse. It is the author's opinion, therefore, that these lesions should be treated at a later stage (after 6 weeks), when the neck fracture has healed, allowing adequate reduction and stabilization of the dislocation (Fig. 10).

3   Group III: Subscapularis Transfer (McLaughlin or Neer's Modification)

When the dislocation is between 4 weeks and 6 months old, or when the McLaughlin lesion has affected more than 25% but less than 40–50% of the humeral head with a history of less than 6 months, McLaughlin's procedure (12) or Neer's modification (3,10) are the best surgical options. Controversy still exists regarding when an arthroplasty should be performed based on the size of the McLaughlin lesion. Neer (7) felt that 50% involvement indicates the need for arthroplasty; Hawkins (10) considers lesions with 40–50% of involvement as the limit; Rockwood (13) considers lesions greater than 40%; and Mestdagh (14) considers a 35% involvement of the humeral head as the limit.

Some authors have proposed that the bone defects in these cases should be treated with associated bone graft fixed with screws. We have treated 12 shoulders (11 patients) with McLaughlin's lesions involving greater than 40% of the articular

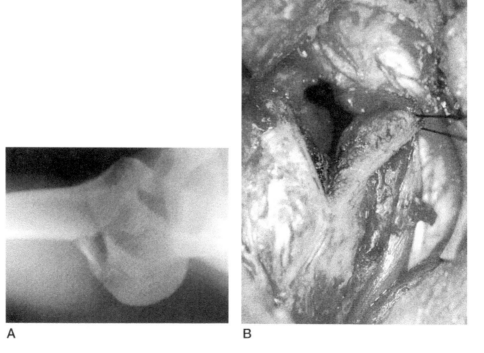

A   B

Figure 9   Example of a locked posterior dislocation associated with fracture of the anatomical neck: (A) axillary view; (B) mini-incision of the subscapularis tendon of the right shoulder showing an empty joint; (C) delicate reduction of the humeral head with a clamp; (D and E) 5-year follow-up x-ray and final elevation.

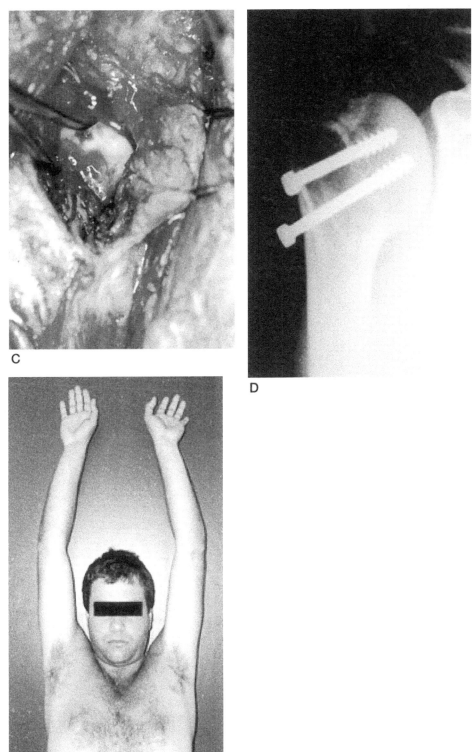

C

D

E

Figure 9 Continued.

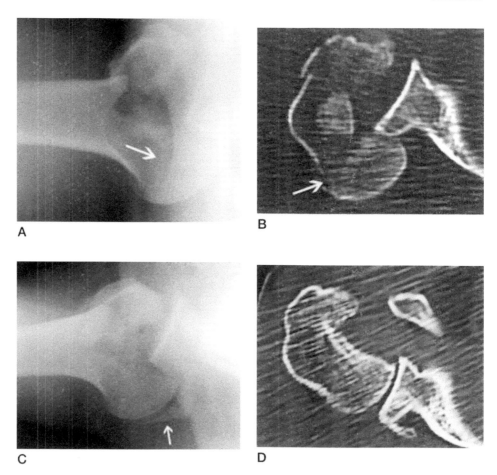

A

B

C

D

Figure 10 X-ray of a locked posterior dislocation with a McLaughlin lesion involving ∼50% of the humeral head associated with a nondisplaced fracture of the anatomical neck. (A) Axillary view, white arrow showing the site of the non-displaced fracture of the anatomical neck; (b) CT scan with a better view of the anatomical neck fracture (white arrow); (c) axillary view 6 weeks after lesion; the white arrow shows the periosteal reaction at the posterior border of the glenoid; (d) 6-year follow-up CT scan showing the large McLaughlin lesion; (E–G) the clinical outcome.

surface with McLaughlin's original technique. At a mean follow-up period of 60 months (range, 12–158 months) (Fig. 10), the only unsatisfactory result was in a noncompliant patient who developed an infection. The mean postoperative range of motion was 140° of elevation, 58° of external rotation, and internal rotation to the T11 level. Postoperative immobilization is required in these cases, and we prefer using a gunslinger type orthosis to keep the shoulder in a fixed position of flexion, abduction, and slight external rotation.

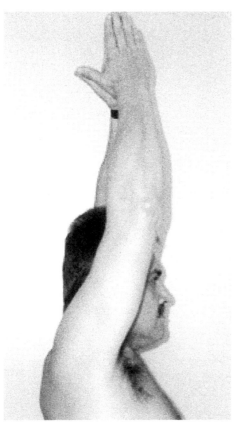

E

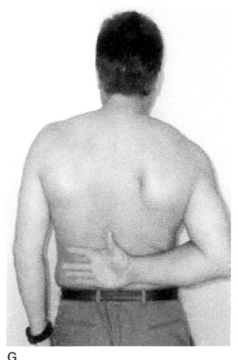

G

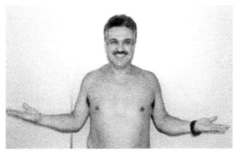

F

Figure 10   Continued.

4   Group IV-A: Hemiarthroplasty in Acute Cases

When lesions of the humeral head are greater than 50%, hemiarthroplasty is the
treatment of choice. Patients who suffer a three-, four-part, and anatomical neck
locked posterior dislocation are candidates for an immediate arthroplasty. In our
series, 5 patients with anatomical neck fractures and one with a four-part fracture
underwent hemiarthroplasty. The procedure was performed with a mean 18.3° of
retroversion of the prosthesis. This is in accordance with Hawkins et al. (10), who
recommended retroversion of 20° in lesions of less than 6 months duration. Caution
must again be taken, however, in that too little retroversion (increased anteversion)
can lead to anterior instability. Soft tissue balancing is critical to maximize outcomes
in these difficult cases.

Our results treating acute cases with arthroplasty have been disappointing.
Only 2 patients had good results. The remaining 3 patients had unsatisfactory results
(2 fair and 1 poor). There are few reports in the literature on the treatment of acute
locked posterior dislocations with hemiarthroplasty. Walch et al. (15) performed
only one hemiarthroplasty in the 30 patients reported in his series. Santos (16)
reported 4 cases, only one of whom had a good result. Neer (7) reported 3 cases with
locked posterior dislocations associated with humeral neck fractures where a
hemiarthroplasty was performed with satisfactory results.

5   Group IV-B: Hemiarthroplasty in Chronic Cases

Hemiarthroplasty is also indicated for chronic lesions older than 6 months and with
preserved glenoid joint cartilage, regardless of the size of the McLaughlin lesion.
Arthroplasty in these cases is technically challenging and requires considerable
surgical skill. Obtaining a balance between stability and mobility is a difficult task.
The subscapularis muscle is usually retracted, and its release is of utmost importance.
One must, however, be very careful to avoid its denervation because the entry points
of the nerves are quite close to the border of the glenoid (17). The next step is the
reduction of the humeral head. Sometimes this reduction is almost impossible, and
Hawkins has suggested removing the humeral head in fragments (10). Following the
osteotomy of the humeral head, a posterior capsuloplasty is sometimes necessary in
order to improve the final stability. This may be done through an anterior approach
(3). The humeral component should be placed in lesser retroversion than that of the
acute cases, between 10 and 20° (10). When the prosthesis has a modular eccentric
head it may be placed with a more anterior offset. Even after performing all of these
technical details, postoperative immobilization in ER for 3–4 weeks is sometimes
recommended in order to obtain a stable arthroplasty.

6   Group V: Total Shoulder Replacement

When degeneration of the cartilage of the glenoid cavity has taken place, a total
shoulder replacement is appropriate. Hawkins (3) felt that lesions occur to the
cartilage approximately 12 months after the dislocation. Total shoulder replacement
is even more technically challenging in this situation than hemiarthroplasty. There
are severe muscular and tendon contractures; the posterior structures are very
stretched and the anterior structures are shortened. Sometimes erosions of the
posterior border of the glenoid must be corrected with bone grafts or even
modification of glenoid version by drilling its anterior edge. After cementing the

glenoid prosthesis, the humeral component should be placed in lesser retroversion than usual (3).

In our experience, 5 out of 6 cases treated with total shoulder replacement had a poor outcome. The mean UCLA score was 17 points, and only one case was classified as good. Neer (18) reported 41 cases of total shoulder replacement for treatment of old fracture-dislocations or malunions of the proximal humerus, obtaining 16 excellent results, 7 satisfactory, and 12 failures; 6 cases with severe lesions were excluded. It is important to stress the great technical difficulties imposed by adherences, soft tissue retraction, and poor bone stock (Fig. 11b).

7 Group VI: Arthrodesis, Resection Arthroplasty, and Rehabilitation

The technical difficulties of the arthroplasty are directly related to the duration of time from the injury to the diagnosis and treatment (19). Sometimes arthrodesis may be the only viable option, but keep in mind that Neviaser (20) stated the older the lesion, the worse the prognosis, regardless of treatment. Hawkins (10) concluded that a total shoulder in patients with locked posterior dislocations is extremely difficult, but felt that this is still the technique that provides the best opportunity for a good functional outcome. Although we agree with Hawkins, when dislocations are over 2 years old, other options should be considered, such as arthrodesis and resection arthroplasty. These techniques can also be used when other treatment options for locked posterior dislocations have failed (Fig. 12).

E. Postoperative Rehabilitation

Radiographs are obtained in all cases at 1, 3, and 6 weeks postoperatively. In addition, radiographs should be made yearly following arthroplasty to check the status of the prosthesis and identify any signs of early failure (lysis, change of position, glenoid wear).

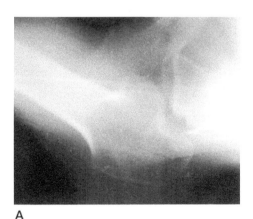
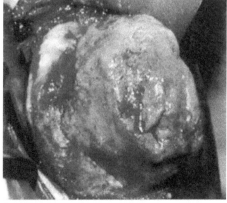

A   B

Figure 11 Preoperative x-ray of a 7-year-old locked posterior dislocation treated with a total shoulder who had an unsatisfactory result. (A) Note the large erosion of the posterior border of the glenoid and the deformity of the humeral head; (B) surgical aspect of the humeral head showing great degeneration of the cartilage.

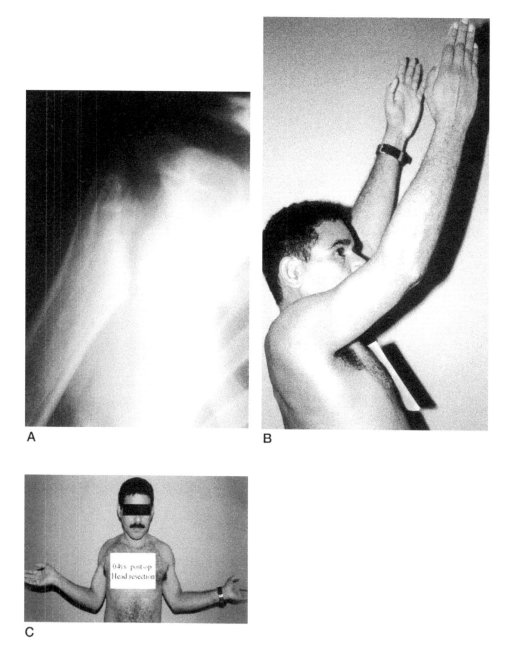

A

B

C

Figure 12   This patient initially underwent total shoulder replacement for locked posterior dislocation but at 4-year follow-up had an unsatisfactory result. The patient then underwent a resection arthroplasty. (A) Four-year postoperative x-ray; (B and C) function.

The specific recommendations for therapy are based on the procedure performed, the stability of the joint, and the quality of the soft tissues. In general, the duration of immobilization usually ranges from 4 to 6 weeks after the McLaughlin or Neer procedure. Patients with longer-standing dislocations are immobilized for 6 weeks, and those with shorter-duration chronic dislocations are immobilized for 4–5 weeks. If there is any concern about stiffness developing, then earlier mobilization may be necessary, and careful weekly evaluation is therefore critical.

IV PEARLS AND PITFALLS

There are many factors that can optimize the outcome following the treatment of locked anterior and posterior dislocations. Determining the time from injury to diagnosis is critically important. In cases of alcoholism or other psychiatric conditions, the dislocation may be chronic and the patient unaware of the diagnosis. Subtle radiographic findings such as soft tissue calcification, blunt, rounded-off bony edges from an old fracture, or periosteal new bone formation may provide insight. In addition, patients who have no pain with attempted range of motion of a fixed dislocated shoulder may well have a chronic dislocation. These cases are dealt with on an individual basis, but nonoperative treatment is often the best option for these patients.

When operative treatment is indicated, attention to soft tissue deformities is vitally important in achieving good functional outcomes. The longer the delay in diagnosis, the greater the soft tissue deformities. Therefore, with chronic dislocations, the difficulty is achieving soft tissue balance, and this factor is responsible for many of the poor outcomes that have been reported in the literature. With increased awareness of this problem and increased modularity in shoulder prostheses, however, we feel that these chronic cases can be successfully treated with arthroplasty.

V SUMMARY

There are several treatment options for locked posterior dislocations that will depend on the associated bone lesions and especially on the time elapsed between the dislocation and the surgical intervention. One must always bear in mind that nonoperative intervention may be the best option in some patients. Function can be surprisingly good in patients with untreated, locked posterior dislocations. These are usually patients that have had their shoulders dislocated for some time and have adapted to the situation.

REFERENCES

1. Cooper A. On the dislocation of the Os humeri upon the dorsum scapular, and upon fractures near the shoulder joint. Guy's Hosp Rep 1839; 4:265–284.
2. McIlveen SJ, Duralde XA. Isolated nerve injuries about the shoulder. In: Bigliani LU, ed. Complications of Shoulder Surgery. Baltimore: Williams & Wilkins, 1993:214–239.
3. Hawkins RJ. Unrecognized dislocations of the shoulder. Instr Course Lect 1985; 34:258–263.

4. Gerber C. Chronic, locked anterior and posterior dislocations. In: Warner JJP, Iannotti JP, Gerber C, eds. Complex and Revision Problems in Shoulder Surgery. Philadelphia: Lippincott-Raven, 1997:99–113.

5. Deliz ED, Flatow EL. Chronic unreduced shoulder dislocations. In: Bigliani LU, ed. Complications of Shoulder Surgery. Baltimore: Williams & Wilkins, 1993:127–138.

6. Checchia SL, Santos PD, Miyazaki AN, Bauer G, Akkari M, Acero EJ. Luxação anterior inveterada de ombro. Rev Bras Ortop 1996; 8:663–669.

7. Neer CS. Displaced proximal humeral fractures. J Bone Joint Surg 1970; 52A:1077–1089.

8. Checchia SL, Santos PD, Miyazaki AN. Surgical treatment of acute and chronic posterior fracture-dislocation of the shoulder. J Shoulder Elbow Surg 1998; 7(1):53–65.

9. Goldman A, Sherman O, Price A, Minkoff J. Posterior fracture dislocation of the shoulder with biceps tendon interposition. J Trauma 1987; 27:1083–1086.

10. Hawkins RJ, Neer CS, Pianta RM, Mendoza FX. Locked posterior dislocation of the shoulder. J Bone Joint Surg 1987; 69A:9–18.

11. Dubousset J. Luxation postérieures de l'epaule. Rev Chir Orthop 1967; 53:65–85.

12. McLaughlin HL. Posterior dislocation of the shoulder. J Bone Joint Surg 1952; 34A:584–590.

13. Rockwood CA. Fractures and dislocations of the shoulder. Part 2: Dislocations about the shoulder. In: Rockwood CA, Green DP, eds. Fractures. Philadelphia: Lippincott, 1975:686–718.

14. Mestdagh H, Urvoy P, Berger M, Perlinski S, Maynou C. Résultats du traitement des luxations postérieurs traumatiques de l'epaule. Rev Chir Orthop 1991; 70:164.

15. Walch G, Boileau P, Martin B, Dejour H. Luxations et fractures-luxations postérieures invétérées de l'epaule: apropós de 30 cas. Rev Chir Orthop 1990; 76:546–548.

16. Santos PS, Bonamin C, Sobania LC. Luxações e fraturas-luxações posteriores fixas do ombro. Rev Bras Ortop 1992; 27:675–680.

17. Checchia SL, Santos PD, Martins MG, Meireles FS. Subscapularis muscle enervation: the effect of arm position. J Shoulder Elbow Surg 1996; 5(3):214–218.

18. Neer CS, Watson KC, Staton FL. Recent experience in total shoulder replacement. J Bone Joint Surg 1982; 64A:319–337.

19. Neer CS. Prosthetic replacement of the humeral head: indications and operative technique. Surg Clin North Am 1963; 43:1581–1597.

20. Neviaser JS. Posterior dislocation of the shoulder: diagnosis and treatment. Surg Clin North Am 1963; 43:1623–1630.

12

Classification and Operative Treatment of Scapula and Glenoid Fractures

MICHAEL D. STOVER and GUIDO MARRA

Loyola University Medical Center, Maywood, Illinois, U.S.A.

I INTRODUCTION

Scapula and glenoid fractures are the least common osseous injuries involving the shoulder girdle (1,2,19). The scarcity is a result of the mobility of the scapulothoracic articulation and the substantial soft tissue envelope surrounding the shoulder. The majority of these fractures are minimally displaced and managed nonoperatively. Due to the relative rarity of the more severely displaced injuries, it is difficult for any individual or institution to gain significant experience in their operative management. As a result, the indications for the operative management of these injuries remain poorly defined and an area of ongoing research. This chapter will focus on the operative techniques used in the management of these uncommon, challenging injuries.

II PREOPERATIVE PLANNING

A Patient Evaluation

The majority of scapula fractures are the result of high-energy trauma. They usually occur from direct trauma, but in the case of some intra-articular fractures, as the result of glenohumeral dislocation (1,5,21), fractures rarely occur in isolation and are associated with multiple osseous and soft tissue injuries, some of which can be life threatening (Table 1) (1,2,14,15,19,23). The mortality rate from these associated injuries has been reported to be as high as 16% (21).

Table 1 Injuries Associated with Scapula Fractures

Osseus	Soft tissue
Rib fractures	Hemopneumothorax
Clavicular fracture	Pulmonary contusion
Skull fracture	Head injury
Spine fractures	Vascular injury
	Brachial plexus injury

Initial management of patients with scapula fractures should follow the standard advanced trauma life-support protocols assessing and managing airway, breathing, and circulation. After patient stabilization, associated injuries are identified and addressed according to their level of importance. Management of scapula fractures is often delayed, as it remains a lower priority in the trauma setting.

The physical examination of the shoulder should begin with inspection of the skin for abrasions and lacerations. Severe abrasions are frequently present, and when the dermal injury is deep, alterations in planned skin incisions are required. A detailed neurological examination should be performed in all alert patients with specific documentation of axillary, musculocutaneous, and suprascapular nerve function. Vascular evaluation should include the brachial and radial artery. When injury is suspected, vascular consultation should be obtained.

Radiographic assessment should include evaluation of the admission chest radiograph and specific shoulder films. Scapula fractures are frequently identified as an incidental finding on the initial admission chest radiograph. These films should be screened for ipsilateral clavicle fractures, rib fractures, and lung injuries. The lateral displacement of the medial border of both scapulae should be determined in relation to the spine. If the affected shoulder is displaced laterally or is associated with a distracted clavicle fracture, significant neurovascular injury should be suspected. These patients require serial vascular evaluations or angiography and a detailed evaluation of the brachial plexus.

An initial radiographic series of the shoulder includes an antero-posterior radiograph in the scapular plane, a scapular outlet view, and an axillary view, which allow assessment of fracture displacement (Fig. 1). When fracture patterns are complex or are intra-articular, computed tomography scanning is performed. Three-dimensional reconstructions can also provide clear visualization of fracture morphology and displacement (Fig. 2).

B Fracture Classification

Scapular fractures are broadly classified as intra-articular and extra-articular fractures. Wilber and Evans (22) demonstrated that the vast majority of these fractures are extra-articular. Forty-five percent of scapular fractures involve the scapular body, 25% the glenoid neck, 10% the glenoid fossa, 8% the acromion, 7% the coracoid process, and 5% the scapular spine. Ideberg further classified glenoid fossa fractures in 1984 (14). Fractures are classified into five types: type I, avulsion of the anterior margin; type II, transverse fracture, which exits inferiorly; type III,

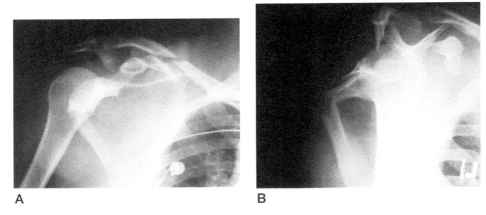

A   B

Figure 1 Initial radiographs include an anteroposterior radiograph (A) and outlet view (B).

oblique fracture through the glenoid, which exits superiorly and is often associated with an acromioclavicular joint injury; type IV, transverse fracture exiting the medial border of the scapula; and type V, a combination of types II and IV.

This system was later modified by Goss, who further subdivided type I fractures: type Ia has involvement of the anterior rim and type Ib has involvement of the posterior rim. Type VI has multiple fracture fragments of the glenoid fossa (9) (Fig. 3).

C Operative Indications

1 Extra-Articular Fractures

Recommendations for the treatment of displaced extra-articular fractures are varied due to the fracture diversity and the small number of reported series (8,10,12,13,17). Fractures involving the glenoid neck with more than 1 cm of displacement and greater than 40° of angulation have been reported to be associated with inferior functional results when managed without operative reduction (1,23). However, recent studies of ipsilateral clavicle and glenoid neck fractures have demonstrated that satisfactory patient outcome can be obtained with both operative and nonoperative treatment (6,7,20). Clear guidelines for operative management of glenoid neck fractures are lacking. The decision for operative management should be based on the degree of fracture displacement, fracture angulation, arm dominance, age, the presence of ipsilateral clavicle fracture, and activity level of the patient.

Operative management of acromial fractures is performed when fracture displacement and angulation compromises the subacromial space. Coracoid fractures require operative fixation only when severe displacement is present in the athlete or in patients with high functional demand.

2 Intra-articular Glenoid Fractures

The main goals in managing glenoid rim and complex intra-articular fractures of the glenoid fossa are restoration of articular congruity and maintenance of glenohumeral stability (3,18). Indications for operative reduction of glenoid rim fractures

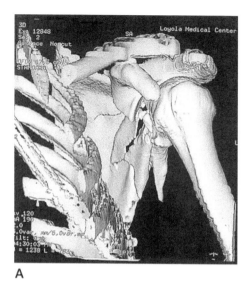

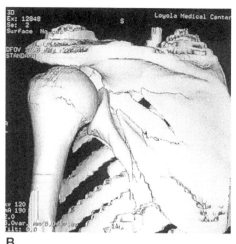

Figure 2 In complex intra-articular fractures three-dimensional reconstruction provides a clear picture of fracture morphology and displacement: (A) anterior view; (B) posterior view; (C) glenoid fossa view with humerus removed.

include fragments involving greater than 25% of the anterior rim, 33% of the posterior rim, or fracture displacement greater than 5 mm.

With complex intra-articular fractures (Ideberg II–VI), open reduction and internal fixation (ORIF) is performed when greater than 5 mm of intra-articular displacement is present. Lesser amounts of displacement may be addressed directly or indirectly in conjunction with operative stabilization of unacceptably displaced fractures of the scapular body or neck.

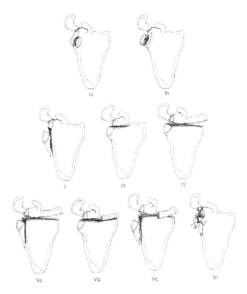

Figure 3 Ideberg classification for intra-articular fractures of the scapula. Type I: avulsion of the anterior margin. Type II: transverse fracture which exits inferiorly. Type III: oblique fracture through the glenoid which exits superiorly and is often associated with an AC injury. Type IV: transverse fracture exiting the medial border of the scapula. Type V is a combination of types II and IV. Type VI is gross comminution of the glenoid fossa. (From Ref. 11.)

III OPERATIVE APPROACH

Operative management of scapula fractures requires a clear preoperative understanding of fracture morphology. Proper instrumentation and selection of operative approach is required for successful management.

A Instrumentation

Instruments required for the operative treatment of scapular fractures include standard small and mini-fragment instrumentation. Plate options include 2.7 and 3.5 mm reconstruction plates, which allow the plates to be contoured to the complex bony anatomy of the scapula. Kirschner wires are needed to provide provisional or definitive fixation of fracture fragments. Cannulated screws and suture anchors should be available for all cases with intra-articular extension. Finally, a radiolucent table and C-arm intensification are used to assess fracture reduction intraoperatively.

B Approaches

The choice of surgical approach is dependent on the fracture location. Four surgical approaches are used to manage scapula fractures: the posterior approach, the anterior approach, the superior approach, and a combined approach (Table 2).

Table 2 Surgical Approaches to Manage Scapula Fractures

Approach	Patient position	Fracture pattern
Anterior	Beach chair	Anterior glenoid rim Coracoid
Posterior	Prone	Posterior glenoid rim Glenoid neck
Superior	Beach chair	Acromion
Combined	Lateral decubitus	Complex intra-articular

1 Posterior Approach

Glenoid Neck and Posterior Rim Fractures.   The posterior approach is reserved for extra-articular fractures that involve the glenoid neck or posterior glenoid rim. Two variations of this approach are described: a muscle-sparing approach and the more extensile Judet approach. The muscle-sparing approach is used when the fracture is isolated to the glenoid neck or to the posterior glenoid rim (4). In more complex fracture patterns, the Judet approach provides excellent visualization of the scapular body, scapular spine, glenoid neck, and the posterior glenoid rim (16).

Patients are placed in the prone position on a radiolucent table with the extremity draped free. Prone positioning facilitates fracture reduction and fixation. However, when significant chest wall or parenchymal lung injuries are present, the lateral decubitus position is preferred to optimize intraoperative ventilation.

The muscle-sparing approach is made with an incision that extends from the posterolateral corner of the acromion distally to the axillary fold (Fig. 4). The medial border of the deltoid is identified and mobilized to expose the underlying infraspinatus and teres minor. Placing the arm in abduction facilitates deltoid retraction and aids in visualization of the underlying structures. The axillary nerve is identified as it exits posteriorly through the quadrilateral space and protected. The interval between the teres minor and infraspinatus is then developed to expose the lateral border of the scapula and posterior inferior glenoid rim. In glenoid neck fractures, this anatomy is often distorted due to the anterior and medial displacement of the articular segment.

The skin incision for the more extensile Judet approach curves from the posterolateral corner of the acromion along the spine of the scapula. It is then carried distally to the inferior angle of the scapula (Fig. 5). The posterior deltoid is sharply detached from the spine of the scapula and reflected laterally exposing the underlying infraspinatus and teres minor. The infraspinatus is then detached from the medial scapular border and reflected laterally on its neurovascular pedicle. This provides excellent exposure of the scapular spine, base of acromion, lateral scapular border, the scapular body, and glenoid neck.

Glenoid Neck Fractures.   The reduction of glenoid neck fractures is greatly facilitated by the prone position. The articular segment is typically displaced in an anterior, medial and inferior direction. Initially, a Schanz pin is placed in the inferior aspect of the posterior glenoid rim. With lateral traction on the arm, reduction can be obtained by manipulation of the Schanz pin. This reduction is held while

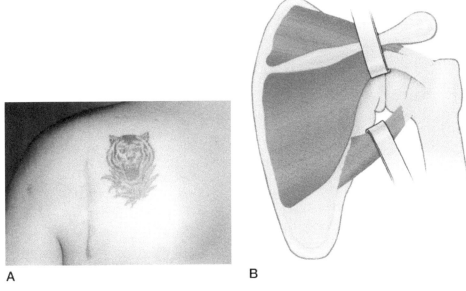

A   B

Figure 4 Posterior surgical exposures: muscle sparing. This approach is reserved for isolated glenoid neck fractures and posterior glenoid rim fractures. (A) Incision extends from the postero-lateral aspect of the acromion caudally. (B) Deep dissection develops the plane between the infraspinatus and teres minor.

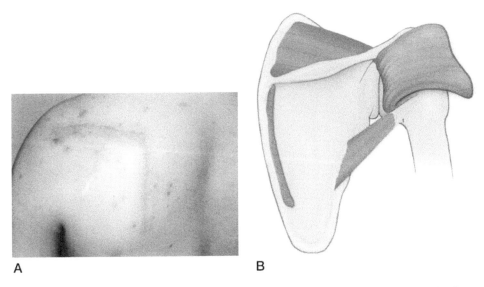

A   B

Figure 5 Posterior surgical exposures: Judet approach. (A) The incision extends along the scapular spine to the medial border of the scapular body. (B) In the deep dissection the infraspinatus is elevated from the medial scapular border and reflected laterally on its neurovascular pedicle. This provides excellent exposure of the scapular body, scapular spine, glenoid neck, and posterior glenoid rim.

provisional fixation is obtained with Kirschner wires passed through the posterior aspect of the acromion into the glenoid neck from a superior approach. Reduction is confirmed with intraoperative fluoroscopy. The Schanz pin is then removed to facilitate plate contouring. A 2.7 or 3.5 mm reconstruction plate is then contoured and fixed along the lateral scapular border and the glenoid neck. Fluoroscopy is used to evaluate the final position of the fracture fragment and to recognize intra-articular screw penetration.

Posterior Rim Fractures. Posterior glenoid rim fractures are visualized by performing a glenoid based T-capsulotomy. Visualization of the glenoid fossa is limited from a posterior approach and requires the use of a humeral head retractor. Direct reduction is obtained and fixation is achieved with two 2.7 or 3.5 mm screws, depending on the size of the posterior rim fragment. Following repair, a careful inspection of the posterior glenoid labrum is performed. When the labrum is detached, suture anchors are used for repair.

2 Anterior Approach

Anterior Glenoid Rim and Coracoid Fractures. The anterior approach is reserved for anterior glenoid rim fractures and coracoid fractures. Patients are placed in a beachchair position with several towels placed under the medial aspect of the scapula to protract and stabilize the scapula. A standard deltopectoral approach is performed with identification and protection of the cephalic vein. The clavipectoral fascia is incised lateral to the conjoined tendon. Often a significant hematoma lies just beneath this fascia, which is evacuated to prevent postoperative scarring. The axillary and musculocutaneous nerves are identified by palpation and direct visualization.

Anterior Glenoid Rim. The subscapularis tendon is identified and divided 2 cm lateral to the musculotendinous junction and dissected from the underlying joint capsule. A retractor is then placed beneath the subscapularis and along the anterior glenoid neck. A glenoid based T-capsulotomy is performed and the humeral head is retracted posteriorly.

The rim fracture is identified and reduced under direct visualization. When a single coronal rim fragment is present, it is anatomically reduced and provisionally fixed with Kirschner wires. Final fixation is achieved with one or two 2.7 or 3.5 mm screws. If the rim fragment can only hold one screw, fixation should be augmented with the use of suture anchor fixation through the labrum above and below the fracture site. When comminution precludes screw fixation, the fragment should be excised. A capsulolabral reconstruction is performed. When greater than 25% of the glenoid fossa is affected, a coracoid transfer is performed to augment the anterior inferior glenoid bone stock.

Corcoid. Fixation of coracoid fractures is performed with a single screw placed through the fragment into the base of the coracoid. When fragmentation prevents screw placement, heavy nonabsorbable suture is placed in the conjoined tendon using a Krackow stitch. The sutures are then passed through drill holes placed on the superior aspect of the coracoid and tied.

3 Superior Approach

The superior approach is used for exposure of acromial fractures. An incision is made parallel to the lateral border of the acromion. Skin flaps are elevated, and the anterior deltoid and coracoacromial ligament are detached from the anterior aspect of the acromion. A split between the anterior and middle deltoid is carried laterally for no more than 4 cm.

The acromial fracture is reduced and fixed with two cannulated screws. This fixation is supplemented with a dorsal tension band performed by passing 18-gauge wire through the screws. Care must be taken to insure that the wires are properly buried in the soft tissues about the shoulder (Fig. 6).

4 Combined Approach

Combined approaches are reserved for the more complex fracture patterns, which involve the glenoid fossa and scapular body. Patients are positioned in a lateral decubitus position to allow for simultaneous anterior and posterior approaches. The major difficulty in these cases is overcoming the deforming force of the humeral head on the fractured glenoid articular surface. Additional assistants are required in these cases to provide lateral arm traction and assist in reduction maneuvers.

The operative approach in these cases requires the anterior and posterior approach as previously described. The anterior approach is used to inspect the glenoid fossa and determine the size and position of the intra-articular fracture. The intra-articular fracture line is lavaged to remove any fragmented bone that can prevent reduction. Reconstruction of the articular surface is obtained by a provisional reduction of the extra-articular component of the fracture through the posterior incision. Through the anterior approach, the intra-articular extension of the fracture is evaluated. Anatomical reduction of this component of the fracture often requires a coordinated reduction maneuver performed through both incisions.

Provisional fixation is obtained with Kirschner wires passed through the acromion. Plates are contoured and applied to the glenoid neck and lateral scapular border. Interfragmentary fixation is obtained by placement of a percutaneous screw from the superior aspect of the glenoid or through the base of the coracoid. When

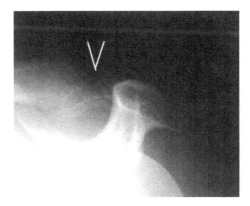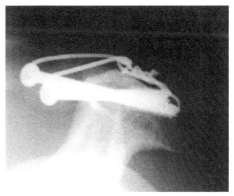

Figure 6 Preoperative and postoperative radiographs of a displaced acromial fracture.

the screw is placed through the base of the coracoid, an incision is made 1 cm anterior and 2–3 cm medial to the acromioclavicular joint. A guide wire for a cannulated screw is placed through the base of the coracoid and passed through to the posterior cortex of the glenoid neck (Fig. 7). When the screw is to be placed through the superior aspect of the glenoid, a skin incision is made just posterior and 1 cm medial to the acromioclavicular joint and passed into the inferior glenoid neck. Confirmation of screw placement is made both by direct intraoperative observation and fluoroscopic imaging.

IV PEARLS AND PITFALLS

The greatest difficulty encountered in the management of scapular injuries involves reduction of the complex intra-articular fractures (Ideburg II–VI). A complete understanding of the fracture is required prior to the operation. In addition, understanding the deforming forces of the dominant fractures fragments is essential in obtaining and maintaining an anatomical reduction. Fractures of the superior glenoid fossa are deformed by the pull of the conjoined tendon and can be tethered by the coracoacromial ligament.

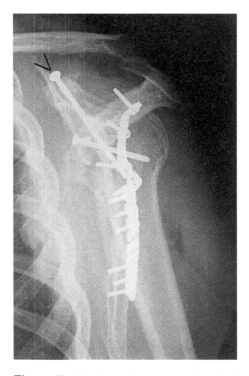

Figure 7 Radiograph demonstrating fixation of a glenoid fossa fracture through the base of the coracoid. The skin incision for this screw is made 1 cm anterior and 2–3 cm medial to the acromioclavicular joint.

Inferior glenoid fossa fractures are deformed by the pull of the triceps tendon. The greatest deforming force remains the weight of the arm transmitted through the articular surface by the humeral head.

Glenoid neck fractures associated with ipsilateral clavicle fracture requiring operative treatment are initially approached with reduction and fixation of the clavicle fracture. Intra-operative radiographs are used to assess the glenoid neck displacement as indirect reduction of the glenoid neck can often be obtained by fixation of the clavicle alone. If unacceptable displacement persists, subsequent ORIF of the scapula fractures is performed.

The version of the glenoid fossa can be difficult to determine intraoperatively from a posterior approach, particularly in the prone position. The tendency will be to reduce the glenoid fossa in excessive anteversion. Proper plate contouring and intraoperative fluoroscopy and/or radiographs are required to confirm glenoid version.

V POSTOPERATIVE REHABILITATION

Cryotherapy is used for the first 48 hours to decrease soft-tissue swelling and assist in pain control. Physiotherapy is initiated on the first postoperative day. The patient and family are instructed on passive elevation and external rotation exercises. The use of narcotic and anti-inflammatory medication is often needed to facilitate early range of motion. At 4 weeks, radiographs are obtained and active assisted range-of-motion and isometric strengthening exercises are instituted. External support is discontinued and functional activities are allowed at 6 weeks. Radiographs are repeated at 8 weeks, and if no displacement is noted, a resistive strengthening program begins.

VI CONCLUSION

Scapula fractures are often minimally displaced and amenable to nonoperative treatment. However, they can serve as a signal for more significant, life-threatening injuries. When significant displacement of intra-articular or extra-articular glenoid fractures is present, careful preoperative evaluation and operative treatment can yield satisfactory clinical results.

REFERENCES

1. Ada JR, Miller ME. Scapular fractures. Analysis of 113 cases. Clin Orthop 1991; 174–180.
2. Armstrong CP, Van der SJ. The fractured scapula: importance and management based on a series of 62 patients. Injury 1984; 15:324–329.
3. Bigliani LU, Newton PM, Steinmann SP, Connor PM, Mcllveen SJ. Glenoid rim lesions associated with recurrent anterior dislocation of the shoulder. Am J Sports Med 1998; 26:41–45.

4. Brodsky JW, Tullos HS, Gartsman GM. Simplified posterior approach to the shoulder joint. J Bone Joint Surg Am 1987; 69:773–774.

5. DePalma AF. Fractures and fracture-dislocations of the shoulder girdle. In: DePalma AF, ed. Surgery of the Shoulder. 3rd ed. Philadephia: J.B. Lippincott, 1983: 362–371.

6. Edwards SG, Whittle AP, Wood GW. Nonoperative treatment of ipsilateral fractures of the scapula and clavicle. J Bone Joint Surg Am 2000; 82:774–780.

7. Egol KA, Connor PM, Karunakar MA, Sims SH, Bosse MJ, Kellam JF. The floating shoulder: clinical and functional results. J Bone Joint Surg Am 2001; 83:1188–1194.

8. Ganz R, Noesberger B. [Treatment of scapular fractures]. Hefte Unfallheilkd 1975; 59–62.

9. Goss TP. Fractures of the glenoid cavity. J Bone Joint Surg Am. 1992; 74:299–305.

10. Goss TP. Double disruptions of the superior shoulder suspensory complex. J Orthop Trauma 1993; 7:99–106.

11. Goss TP. Scapular fractures and dislocations: diagnosis and treatment. J Acad Am Orthop Surg 1995; 3:22–33.

12. Hardegger FH, Simpson LA, Weber BG. The operative treatment of scapular fractures. J Bone Joint Surg [Br] 1984; 66:725–731.

13. Herscovici D Jr. Open reduction and internal fixation of ipsilateral fractures of the scapular neck and clavicle [letter; comment]. J Bone Joint Surg Am 1994; 76:1112–1113.

14. Ideberg R. Fractures of the scapula involving the glenoid fossa. In: Bateman JE, Welsh RP, eds. Surgery of the Shoulder. Philadelphia: B.C. Decker, 1984; 63–66.

15. Imatani RJ. Fractures of the scapula: a review of 53 fractures. J Trauma 1975; 15:473–478.

16. Judet R. Traitment chirurgical des fractures de l'omoplate. Acta Orthop Belg 1904; 30:673–678.

17. Leung KS, Lam TP. Open reduction and internal fixation of ipsilateral fractures of the scapular neck and clavicle [see comments]. J Bone Joint Surg Am 1993; 75:1015–1018.

18. Mayo KA, Benirschke SK, Mast JW. Displaced fractures of the glenoid fossa. Results of open reduction and internal fixation. Clin Orthop 1998; 122–130.

19. McGahan JP, Rab GT, Dublin A. Fractures of the scapula. J Trauma 1980; 20:880–883.

20. Ramos L, Mencia R, Alonso A, Ferrandez L. Conservative treatment of ipsilateral fractures of the scapula and clavicle. J Trauma 1997; 42:239–242.

21. Thompson DA, Flynn TC, Miller PW, Fischer RP. The significance of scapular fractures. J Trauma 1985; 25:974–977.

22. Wilber MC, Evans EB. Fractures of the scapula. An analysis of forty cases and a review of the literature. J Bone Joint Surg [Am] 1977; 59:358–362.

23. Zdravkovic D, Damholt VV. Comminuted and severely displaced fractures of the scapula. Acta Orthop Scand 1974; 45:60–65.

13

Treatment of Clavicle Fractures and Malunions

CARL J. BASAMANIA

Duke University Medical Center, and Durham Veterans Administration Hospital, Durham, North Carolina, U.S.A.

I INTRODUCTION

The clavicle is a truly eloquent bone. It has a unique shape and is the only long bone in the body to form via intramembranous ossification. It is the first bone to ossify and the last to stop growing. It is the only diarthrodial link between the upper extremity and the rest of the axial skeleton. Even Codman noted that "it seems to me that the clavicle is one of man's greatest skeletal inheritances" in that it sets us off from other animals. It is the most commonly fractured bone in childhood and accounts for about 15% of all fractures and 44% of upper extremity fractures.

II BIOMECHANICS AND FUNCTION

The clavicle provides the only bony link between the thorax and the entire upper extremity. Epiphyseal growth plates develop at both the medial and lateral ends of the bone, but it is the medial ossification center that is responsible for the majority of the longitudinal growth of the bone (approximately 80%). In the upright, resting position, the clavicle is under constant bending load from the force of gravity relentlessly pulling down on the combined mass of the upper extremity and any load carried therein. The area just distal to the subclavius muscle insertion is mechanically the weakest point. This is likely the reason that most fractures of the clavicle occur exactly in this area with uncanny regularity.

Disruption of the middle third of the clavicle will result in depression of the distal segment with the attached upper extremity. The medial segment, when released from its load, will elevate. The sternocleidomastoid pulls the proximal fragment superiorly and posteriorly. The pectoralis major muscle causes shortening at the fracture site and medial rotation of the distal segment and attached upper extremity through its attachments and action on the proximal humerus. The weight of the arm pulls the distal fragment distally. The resultant deformity is multiplanar, and this must be appreciated when treating clavicle fractures (Fig. 1).

Clavicular disruptions anywhere along its length will affect a patient's ability to generate and transmit forces to the upper extremity. Congenital absence of the clavicle as in cleidocranial dysostosis may result in some weakness in supporting overhead loads. Excision of the clavicle invariably results in the shoulder girdle drooping anteriorly and medially. These patients have weakness and pain that can be disabling. Significant shortening of the clavicle as in malunion can result in a vague feeling of "weakness" in the shoulder, especially during overhead activity. Strength testing of the pectoralis major muscle in patients with shortened malunions of the clavicle will demonstrate this finding. The measurable weakness in this muscle group is likely attributable to decreasing the distance between the origin and insertion of the muscle. In addition, there can be a significant change in the orientation of the glenohumeral joint with a clavicle malunion (Fig. 2). Clavicle malunions represent fixed or static anteriomedial displacements of the shoulder, whereas clavicle nonunions are more like acromioclavicular (AC) separations in that they are more dynamic. Some authors have suggested the as much as 15 mm of shortening can lead to poor long-term results and patient dissatisfaction. Nonunion of a clavicle fracture can add another variable to the equation, since the clavicle can be both short and unstable. The instability denies the shoulder girdle muscles of the rigid post against which they generate their force, particularly in the overhead position. A muscle deprived of a stable post to pull against is unable to generate the magnitude of force required for most activities.

Direct trauma by sharp fracture ends, clavicular nonunion, clavicular malunion, or healing with exuberant callus can place any of the structures in the

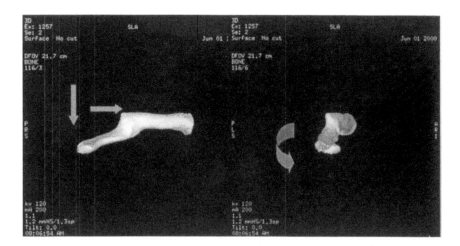

Figure 1 Anteromedial and inferior rotation of the shoulder due to loss of clavicular length in a malunion.

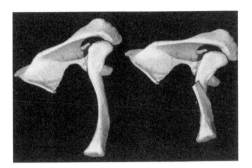

Figure 2 Change in the orientation of the glenoid due to scapular rotation around the thorax which is seen in clavicle fractures.

costoclavicular space at risk, but the most commonly affected is the medial cord and ulnar nerve.

Several large studies of clavicle fractures have been published detailing the apparent mechanism of injury, including falls on the point of the shoulder or onto an outstretched hand. Although rare, serious associated injuries to the great vessels, brachial plexus, or lungs and pleura can occur and may become potentially life threatening.

III RADIOGRAPHIC EVALUATION

The appropriate radiographic evaluation will depend on the site of the clavicle injury and on any associated injuries. Potentially life-threatening associated injuries will obviously take precedence. In the unconscious patient, a chest film and cervical spine films should be the first radiographs completed. A chest film should also be obtained when the history or physical exam suggests possible thoracic injury. An abnormal vascular exam of the upper extremity may require an arteriogram.

Fractures of the middle third of the clavicle are easily imaged; however, a recurrent problem we have encountered is that an anteroposterior (AP) of the shoulder is often the only view obtained in many emergency rooms. Clavicular shaft fractures are generally easy to identify when viewed in an anteroposterior projection centered on the mid-shaft of the clavicle. A 45° cephalic tilt film will more clearly delineate the fracture anatomy, amount of displacement, and extent of comminution (Fig. 3). We routinely obtain an AP and 45° cephalic tilt AP on all clavicle fractures. The typical pattern in a low-energy injury is an oblique fracture. The proximal fragment is displaced superiorly and posterior by the pull of the sternocleidomastoid muscle. The distal fragment is depressed by the weight of the upper extremity. If there is complete displacement of the fracture or comminution, the distal fragment is most commonly pulled medially by the pectoralis major, and thus underrides the proximal fragment. To evaluate the amount of shortening at the fracture site, we recommend an anteroposterior view of both clavicles on a wide cassette including the sternum and the acromioclavicular joints. This x-ray allows fairly accurate measurement of the clavicular lengths.

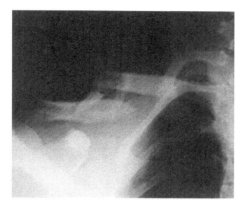

Figure 3 Typical clavicle fracture pattern as seen on 45° cephalic tilt AP radiographs.

Fractures of the distal third of the clavicle are more difficult to image. Standard x-ray technique for either the clavicular shaft or the shoulder overexposes the distal clavicle. Also, a straight AP view of the region obscures the distal clavicle and AC joint in the overlap of the scapula and acromion. Subtle fractures and particularly intra-articular fractures are inadequately displayed using standard techniques. Routine films of this region should include a 15° cephalic tilt AP centered on the AC joint, using soft tissue technique (Zanca view), and an axillary lateral view.

IV TREATMENT GOALS AND OBJECTIVES

The primary goal in clavicle fractures is to obtain solid union of the fracture while at the same time avoiding undue risks of either late or iatrogenic complications. The next goal is to restore function to the injured upper extremity and to allow the patient to return to full activity as soon as possible. In general, there are three options available to achieve the first goal: partial immobilization and support of the upper extremity, closed reduction and partial immobilization, and closed or open reduction and internal fixation. Achieving the second goal may require early application of a rehabilitative protocol and/or sport-specific rehabilitation. This may merely involve maintaining aerobic fitness or instituting a strengthening program designed to maintain strength in the other uninjured extremities.

A Partial Immobilization and Support of the Upper Extremity

This option is preferable when the fracture alignment is acceptable and there are no other indications for reduction or operative fixation of the fracture. Options include sling, sling and swathe, Sayre bandage, Velpeau dressing, and modified Velpeau, to name only a few. If the displacement seen on the initial injury films is acceptable, this method is likely to maintain adequate partial immobilization at the fracture site to allow healing in this position. Functional and cosmetic results can be expected to be essentially the same as that achieved with figure-8 bandages.

B Reduction and Partial Immobilization with or Without Support of the Closed Upper Extremity

Since the proximal fragment cannot be controlled, reduction maneuvers are designed to bring the depressed and medially rotated distal fragment(s) up to and back to the proximal fragment. Various forms of figure-8 bandages both with and without support of the upper extremity have been designed to help achieve this goal. The various figure-8 dressings all require periodic adjustments. Occasionally, patients may be unable to tolerate the dressing secondary to pain at the fracture site or neurovascular compromise while wearing the figure-8 bandages. There is no evidence that a figure-8 bandage or variant provides any better functional or cosmetic result than partial immobilization and support alone. In fact, these studies have found the results to be identical and furthermore unchanged from the initial fracture displacement on the injury films. This suggests that the amount of displacement identified on the initial injury films will determine the ultimate position if union occurs. Thompson noted that a 100% displaced middle third clavicle fracture is at particular risk for nonunion unless bony contact can be achieved and maintained.

Soft tissue interposition was thought to be a major contributing factor in the formation of clavicular nonunion in a study by Manske and Szabo. They found that one of the fragments is frequently impaled in the trapezius muscle. In several acute fractures treated with open reduction and intramedullary fixation, and in two malunions, we found that one of the supraclavicular nerves was entrapped in the fracture site (Fig. 4). In higher energy fracture patterns, we have found soft tissue interposition to be a very frequent finding. However, others have reported that this is uncommon. A reduction maneuver may also be indicated when there is evidence of neurovascular compromise that is persistent or progressive and in cases where the overlying skin is in jeopardy of necrosis.

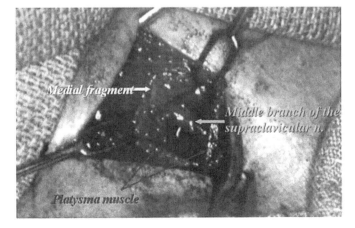

Figure 4 Intraoperative photo showing the middle branch of the supraclavicular nerve under the medial fragment of the clavicle.

C   Closed or Open Reduction and Internal Fixation

The methods available include soft tissue and suture procedures alone, intramedullary devices, plate fixation, external fixation and, for distal clavicle fractures, coracoclavicular screw fixation.

The indications for operative treatment of acute clavicle fractures include:

Open fractures

Medial clavicle fractures, including growth plate injuries with posterior impingement on vital structures and/or causing symptoms such as brachial plexopathy, thoracic outlet syndrome, difficulty swallowing, and difficulty breathing

Neurovascular compromise requiring immediate exploration or that is progressive or unresponsive to closed reduction maneuvers

Displacement severe enough to tent the skin and impair its blood flow, possibly leading to necrosis

The so-called "floating shoulder" combination of fractures

Displaced, comminuted, and shortened fractures of the middle third of the clavicle, particularly in the dominant extremity of the throwing athlete

Patients who, because of job demands, are unable to tolerate a program of prolonged immobilization such as a surgeon, barber, or self-employed worker

Patients unable to tolerate closed treatment, such as patients with Parkinson's, disease seizures, or other ataxias

Distal clavicle fractures that are completely displaced and irreducible with intact coracoclavicular ligaments

Displaced distal clavicle fractures with rupture of the coracoclavicular ligaments

Multitrauma patients, especially ones with lower extremity fractures that require use of the upper extremities for transfers and crutch ambulation

V TREATMENT OPTIONS

A   Medial Clavicle Fractures

These fractures are rare, comprising about 5% of all clavicle fractures in adults. As stated previously, the medial clavicular physis is the last in the body to fuse, occurring between ages 22 and 25. Many medial clavicle fractures are therefore physeal injuries, which inherently have great healing potential. Anterior displacement, even if complete, is not a concern. The great majority of these fractures are best treated nonoperatively with figure-8 bandages or a sling. Healing is usually rapid with a very low risk for nonunion.

The medial clavicle fracture that can be very problematic is that with posterior displacement severe enough to impinge upon the vital structures at the root of the neck. Patients with complaints of difficulty swallowing or breathing or with any neurovascular compromise will require operative reduction of the fracture. Furthermore, patients without symptoms but with documented computed tomography (CT) scan evidence of impingement of the fragments on vital structures should be considered for operative reduction. Reduction maneuvers or a "towel clip" reduction should not be performed in the clinic or the emergency room unless the posterior position of the fragment is causing an airway or hemodynamic emergency. This reduction must be performed in the operating room under general anesthesia. The chest must be prepped as for a sternotomy, and a thoracic surgeon must be available in case there is a vascular problem. A towel clip can be used to grasp the distal fragment and pull it forward to the proximal fragment. Traction on the upper extremity or a towel placed between the shoulder blades may assist in unlocking the fragments and allowing reduction. The reduction is generally stable. In cases where the reduction is unstable or unobtainable, open reduction will be necessary. Removing interposed soft tissue will likely allow reduction and should stabilize the fracture. Fixation may be obtainable with heavy suture and repair of the soft tissue envelope. In some cases plate and screw fixation may be necessary. In these cases the vital structures must be protected beneath the clavicle with a curved retractor to prevent plunging with the drill.

B Middle Third Fractures

The majority of middle third fractures or shaft fractures of the clavicle can be managed best by closed means either with a figure-8 splint or a sling. Reduction maneuvers and figure-8 bandages have not been conclusively shown to hold a reduction or improve cosmesis in these fractures. It has been our experience that even if a "reduction" is obtained, it will almost always revert to the position seen immediately after the injury. Reduction of these fractures seem to be maintained better in children, however. A fracture that is completely displaced and/or severely shortened is likely to stay in this position or revert to this position despite reduction and the tightest figure-8 bandage. The problematic fractures of the mid-shaft of the clavicle are generally those that have absorbed greater energy. In our experience, these higher-energy fractures tend to have a remarkably consistent pattern. They are generally shortened and comminuted with a butterfly fragment that is consistently anterior and inferior. Soft tissue injury and stripping is usually significant, and instability is common. All of these factors increase the risk of nonunion in any fractured bone. We believe that these fractures are best treated with open reduction and internal fixation. Two surgical options include plate and screw fixation and intramedullary fixation.

If plate and screw fixation is chosen, dynamic compression or limited-contact dynamic compression plates should be used. The forces across this bone are too great to tolerate semi-tubular or one-third tubular plates. Although reconstructive plates have been used, there is a higher likelihood that these too can fail, so we do not recommend their use. It is best to obtain at least three screws in each fragment, and preferably six cortices. The exposure must be large enough to allow placement of all these screws, and, much more importantly, the exposure must allow protection of the structures directly beneath the clavicle. This will require the placement of a curved retractor or other protective device beneath the clavicle while drilling the holes. Although plate and screw fixation provides good stability, it requires more soft tissue stripping than intramedullary fixation. This soft tissue stripping may compromise clavicular healing since most, if not all, of the blood supply to the clavicle is periosteal. In active patients, early motion may lead to hardware failure (Fig. 5).

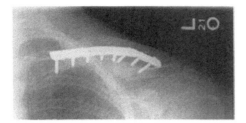

Figure 5   Patient in whom appropriate plate fixation was used; however, there was a loss of fixation in the distal fragment.

Therefore, we prefer intramedullary fixation for most of these fractures using a modified Hagie pin (Depuy Corp). We believe this method to be superior for several reasons. The exposure to place an intramedullary pin is significantly smaller than that needed for a formal open reduction and internal fixation with plates and screws. This limits further damage to the already compromised soft tissue envelope. The intramedullary pin allows for compression at the fracture site and load sharing and is easily removable using local anesthesia. Intramedullary pins come in different sizes allowing proper canal fill, which has been shown to be advantageous in other fractures treated with intramedullary devices. Unlike plate and screw fixation, placement of the intramedullary pin does not require the need to perpendicularly drill through the clavicle. This decreases the risk to the neurovascular structures and obviates the need to strip the soft tissues to allow for protection of these structures. In our experience, we have never seen a subsequent fracture through this region.

C   Clavicle Malunions

There has been very little published on the treatment of malunions of the clavicle. Although most clavicle fractures heal, it is not unusual for prominent callus to form. This has been associated with a number of problems, including compression of the brachial plexus, subclavian vein, and artery and thoracic outlet syndrome. Although numerous case studies have reported complications of clavicle fractures, few studies have examined the long-term sequelae of the fractures themselves. Although most clavicle fractures in adults heal, it is not unusual to have symptoms related to the fracture in a third of adults even 3 months after the injury. In the few studies looking at long-term follow-up after clavicle fractures, Eskola found that patients who had as little as 1.5 cm of shortening tended to have chronic pain. Hill reported that 31% of patients were dissatisfied with the results of nonoperative treatment at an average of 3 years postinjury and initial shortening of >20 mm had a significant association with nonunion and unsatisfactory results.

The two basic problems the surgeon must address in clavicle malunions are the prominent deformity, due to angulation of the fracture fragments, and shortening of the clavicle. Some authors have reported "shaving down" the prominent callus; however, this has resulted in rather dismal results in our experience. Furthermore, this technique does not restore the length of the clavicle. Jupiter reported on a technique used in a small number of patients in whom he osteotomized the clavicle and used a "sculptured" tricortical graft to return the clavicle to its normal length.

The clavicle was then fixed with a plate and screws. Although an attempt was made to return the clavicle to its normal length, a specific attempt to reduce the prominence of the clavicle was not made. Although this restores length to the clavicle, the malunion represents a multiplanar deformity and it is diificult to correct all the planes of deformity with a single osteotomy. An additional potential problem with this technique is the amount of soft tissue stripping required for plating of the clavicle.

D Surgical Technique for Intramedullary Fixation

Step 1: Patient Positioning

Place the patient in a beach chair position on the operating table. Visualization of the clavicle and shoulder access is facilitated by using a radiolucent shoulder-positioning device. An image intensification device or C-arm greatly facilitates pin placement and can help reduce the anxiety that may be associated with drilling the clavicle. Bring the C-arm base in from the head of the bed with the C-arm gantry rotated slightly away from the operative shoulder, oriented with a cephalic tilt. The C-arm can then be draped into the field to decrease the need to bring the C-arm in and out of the field and to allow monitoring the procedure at any point during the case (Fig. 6).

Step 2: Incision

Make a 3-cm incision in Langer's lines over the distal end of the medial fragment (Fig. 7). This is done because the clavicle skin is moved medially more easily than laterally. Most patients have a deep skin crease in the same area where the incision is made. Placing the incision in this crease results in a more cosmetically pleasing scar.

Since little subcutaneous fat is in this region, take care to prevent injury to the underlying platysma muscle. Use scissors to free the platysma muscle from the overlying skin. Once the platysma muscle has been identified, divide its fibers

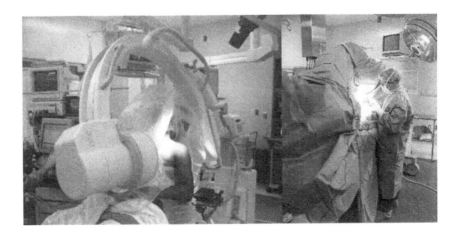

Figure 6 Position of the C-arm for intramedullary fixation of the clavicle. The C-arm can be draped into the field to allow excellent intraoperative imaging of the clavicle without the need for repeatedly bringing the machine over the patient.

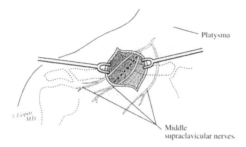

Figure 7 Typical incision with its relationship to the underlying platysma muscle and the middle branch of the supraclavicular nerve.

longitudinally. Also, great care should be used to prevent injury to the middle branch of the supraclavicular nerve, usually found directly beneath the platysma muscle near the midclavicle. Identify and retract the nerve to prevent injury. With acute fractures, the periosteum over the fracture site is disrupted and usually requires no further division. In most cases, there will be interposed muscle and soft tissue. Carefully remove them with an elevator or curette. Leave small butterfly fragments, usually found anteriorly, attached to their soft tissue envelope.

Step 3: Drilling and Tapping the Intramedullary Canal

Elevate the proximal end of the medial clavicle through the incision using a towel clip, elevator, or bone-holding forceps. Since the drills, taps, and intramedullary pins are in sets, use either the smooth end of the taps or the drills to size the canal. Taking care not to penetrate the anterior cortex, drill the intramedullary canal (Fig. 8). The fit should not be too loose as this may compromise fixation or too tight as this may split the bone. The C-arm can be used to check orientation of the drill. Then, remove the drill from the medial fragment and attach the same sized tap to the T-handle and tap the intramedullary canal to the anterior cortex (Fig. 9).

Next, elevate the lateral fragment through the incision. Connect the same sized drill used in the medial fragment to the ratchet T-handle and drill the intramedullary canal. Pass the drill under C-arm guidance out through the posterolateral cortex of the clavicle, which will be posterior to the AC joint (Fig. 10). The drill should

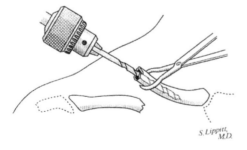

Figure 8 Reaming of the medullary canal of the clavicle using an appropriately sized drill bit.

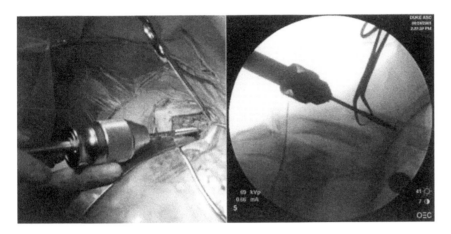

Figure 9 Tapping of the medial fragment.

penetrate the posterolateral cortex at a point just above and slightly lateral to the conoid tubercle. Then, remove the drill from the lateral fragment, attach the same sized tap to the T-handle, and tap the intramedullary canal so that the large threads are advanced fully into the canal (Fig. 8).

Step 4: Insertion of the Clavicle Pin

While still holding the distal fragment with a bone clamp, pass the trocar end of the DePuy clavicle pin into the medullary canal of the distal fragment. The pin should exit through the previously drilled hole in the posterolateral cortex. Once the pin exits the clavicle, its tip can be felt subcutaneously. Make a small incision over the palpable tip and spread the subcuntaneous tissue with a hemostat (Fig. 11). Place the

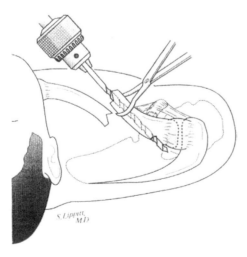

Figure 10 Ideal exit point in the lateral clavicular fragment. The point is just lateral to the conoid tubercle.

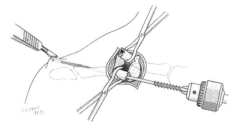

Figure 11   Passage of the clavicle pin through the posterolateral cortex of the clavicle.

tip of the hemostat under the tip of the clavicle pin to facilitate its passage through the incision. Then, drill the pin out laterally until the large, medial threads start to engage the cortex. Attach the Jacobs chuck to the end of the pin protruding laterally and carefully advance the medial end of the clavicle pin into the lateral fragment until only the smooth tip is protruding from the lateral fragment (Fig. 12).

The weight of the arm usually pulls the arm downward; therefore, the shoulder needs to be lifted up to facilitate pin passage into the medial fragment. Place the medial nut on the pin, followed by the smaller lateral nut. Cold weld the two nuts together by grasping the medial nut with a needle driver or needlenose pliers and tightening the lateral nut against the medial nut using the lateral nut wrench (Fig. 13). Reduce the fracture and pass the pin into the medial fragment using the T-handle and wrench on the lateral nut until it comes in contact with the anterior cortex (Fig. 14). This position can be verified by the C-arm or by taking a x-ray.

Step 5:   Securing the Pin

Break the cold weld between the nuts by grasping the medial nut with a needle driver or pliers and quickly turning the lateral nut counterclockwise with the insertion wrench. Advance the medial nut until it is against the lateral cortex of the clavicle.

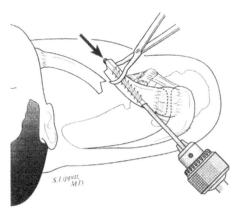

Figure 12   Advancement of the pin into the lateral fragment until only the smooth medial tip of the pin is exposed.

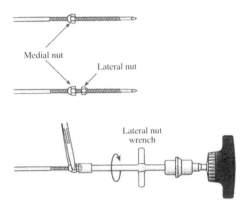

Figure 13   Placement of the medial and lateral nuts on the pin. The offset sizes allow use of an insertion wrench and an extraction wrench for easier insertion and removal of the pin.

Then, tighten the lateral nut until it engages the medial nut. Use the pin cutter to cut the pin near the lateral nut.

Step 6:   Soft Tissue Closure

To reapproximate the anterior butterfly fragments, pass the Crego elevator beneath the clavicle in an anterior-to-posterior direction to protect the underlying structures. Use absorbable Ethicon #0 or #1 PDS or Panacryl sutures loaded on a CTX or CT1 needle and pass it through the periosteum attached to the butterfly fragment. Then, pass it around and beneath the clavicle (Fig. 15). Carefully direct the needle toward the Crego elevator, so it will be deflected by the elevator. Retrieve the needle posteriorly. Pass the suture in a figure-8 manner or use multiple simple sutures to cerclage the butterfly fragment to the main fracture fragments. Close the periosteum overlying the fracture with multiple figure-8 sutures of 0 absorbable suture.

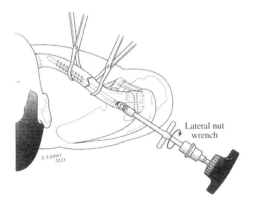

Figure 14   Reduction of the fracture and antegrade passage of the pin into the medial fragment.

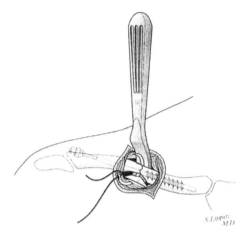

Figure 15 Suture circlage of the anterior butterfly fragment. A Crego elevator is placed beneath the clavicle to prevent damage to the underlying structures and facilitate passage of the needle around the clavicle.

Reapproximate the platysma muscle with simple nonabsorbable Ethicon #2-0 vicryl sutures. Close both incisions with a running subcuticular suture.

E   Postoperative Care of Acute Fractures

Allow the patient to resume daily living activities as soon as tolerated, but avoid strenuous activities such as pulling, lifting or pushing, and arm elevation higher than face level for 4–6 weeks. Excessive arm motion, particularly forward flexion, may result in rotation of the fracture fragments causing irritation of the soft tissue by the lateral pin and nuts. Remove sutures at 7–10 days. Postoperative x-rays should be taken at the 4- to 6-week postoperative clinic visit. If the fracture is clinically healed (nontender, palpable callus), allow the patient to advance daily activities as tolerated. The patient should be seen at 8–12 weeks postoperatively. If repeat x-rays (AP and 45° cephalic tilt AP radiographs) show healing of the fracture, the pin may be removed. This can be done in the clinic or in an ambulatory surgery setting.

F   Pin Removal

The patient is placed in a lateral decubitus positon or in a beach chair position that allows full access to the posterolateral aspect of the involved shoulder. The skin in the area of the previous posterior incision is infiltrated with 1% lidocaine. The previous incision is incised and the lateral wrench is used to retighten the lateral nut to make sure the cold weld is established. The medial wrench is then placed on the medial nut and the pin is removed like a screw (Fig. 16). Care should be taken not to remove the pin too quickly as this may cause the patient discomfort or pin breakage. The wound is closed with a simple subcutaneous absorbable suture. The patient is allowed to advance to full, unrestricted activity over the following month (Fig. 17).

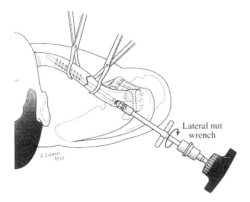

Figure 16 Removal of the clavicle pin using the extraction wrench.

G Optional Technique for Clavicle Malunions and Nonunions

For clavicle malunions, incise the periosteum overlying the deformity longitudinally as previously described. Once the periosteum is circumferentially elevated from the deformity, use a small osteotome to remove the callus from the fracture site. This is best performed under C-arm guidance to assure adequate removal of the fracture callus (Fig. 18). Use a rongeur to remove the callus from the ends of the medial and lateral fracture fragments. Then, find the canal with the smallest size drill bit, verify its position with a C-arm or an x-ray, and then drill the canal with the appropriate size drill. Pass the DePuy clavicle pin as previously noted. Use a small osteotome to "fish scale" the cortical bone about the fracture site. Morsellize the previously removed callus, and pack it around the fracture site (Fig. 19). Autogenous bone graft from the patient should be used when indicated. Then, close the periosteum as previously noted.

Treat hypertrophic nonunions the same as clavicle malunions, taking care to remove all the interposed pseudocapsule. In the case of atrophic nonunions, remove any tapered ends of the clavicle fragments. Carefully remove the scar tissue with a rongeur. Proceed with treatment as described for clavicle malunion, with the exception of using autologous or autograft bone. We have found that patients tolerate autologous bone graft taken from the proximal tibia far better than iliac crest graft. If structural bone is needed, tricortical graft from the crest can be used. If only cancellous graft is necessary, a small incision can be made over the anterior aspect of the tibia just anterior to Gerdy's tubercle. A small cortical window is opened using a 1/4 in. osteotome, and cancellous bone is then taken with a curette. This can be done under local with intravenous sedation and, when combined with regional anesthesia for the clavicle, greatly facilitates the immediate postop recovery.

Postoperative Care

The postoperative care and timing of the pin removal for malunions and nonunions needs to be modified as required. Usually patients can resume full activities of daily living after at least 4 weeks. With clavicle nonunions and malunions, leave the pin in

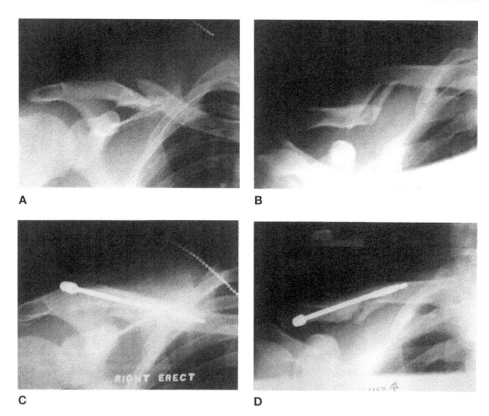

Figure 17 (A–F) Radiographs showing injury, pin placement, and final result of a comminuted clavicle fracture. (G) Clinical result showing well-healed incision.

place for a minimum of 12 weeks, or until there is evidence of good healing on radiographs. Then, remove the pin as previously described. Use both AP and 45° cephalic tilt AP radiographs to assess healing (Fig. 20).

VI DISTAL CLAVICLE FRACTURES

In this section we will consider those fractures that involve or are distal to the conoid tubercle of the clavicle. Fractures that are medial to the conoid tubercle can generally be treated like middle third fractures, but those lateral to the conoid present differing concerns and treatment requirements due to the presence of the coracoclavicular ligaments and their effects on fracture stability.

Nondisplaced fractures of the distal clavicle are best treated with a sling. As symptoms allow, the patient is weaned from the sling and started on a shoulder rehabilitation program. The earliest return to sports activity is generally around 6–8 weeks following the injury. In collision sports, extra padding or a fiberglass "shell" may be necessary to protect the distal clavicle. The patient must be advised that early return to sports involves some risk of refracture or displacement.

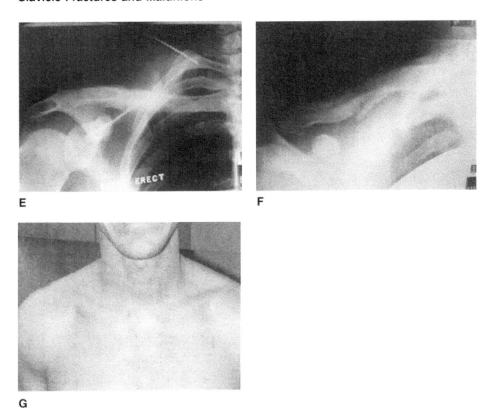

E

F

G

Nondisplaced fractures that involve the acromioclavicular joint deserve special note. The treatment is the same, but it is important to inform the patient that the involvement of the joint increases the likelihood of chronic pain due to posttraumatic acromioclavicular joint arthrosis.

The treatment of displaced distal clavicle fractures hinges on the integrity of the coracoclavicular and acromioclavicular ligaments. More precisely, the treatment generally depends on whether or not the conoid portion of the coracoclavicular ligaments is still attached to the medial fragment of the clavicle. If the conoid ligament remains attached to the medial fragment, it will help prevent large displacement at the fracture site. The fracture fragments should remain relatively close to one another, and this fracture can be expected to heal with sling treatment. When the conoid ligament is disrupted, the distal clavicle fragment with the attached scapula (through AC and CC ligaments) will droop inferiorly and medially under the weight of the attached upper extremity. The medial clavicular fragment, now unencumbered, will elevate away from the distal fragment. This raises the risk for nonunion and chronic medial rotational instability of the shoulder through the fracture site.

Several clues are useful in ascertaining the integrity of the conoid ligament. Often, rupture of the conoid ligament is obvious on x-ray by the fracture occurring lateral to the conoid tubercle with marked increase in the coracoclavicular interval

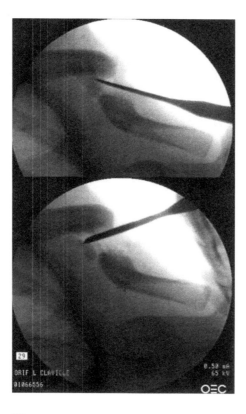

Figure 18 Removal of malunion callus under C-arm guidance.

and marked fracture displacement. It is difficult to discern the integrity when fractures occur at or very near the conoid tubercle. When both CC ligaments are attached to the distal fragment, the fracture line is usually oblique with the CC interval maintained between the coracoid and the distal fragment. There is usually wide fracture displacement. In equivocal cases, medial rotational instability at the

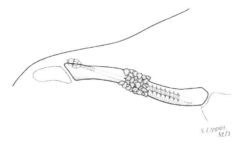

Figure 19 Previously removed callus is morselized and placed about the fracture site after a small osteotome is used to fish-scale the ends of the fragments. Care should be taken not to place too much graft behind or under the clavicle as this may result in compression of the plexus or vessels.

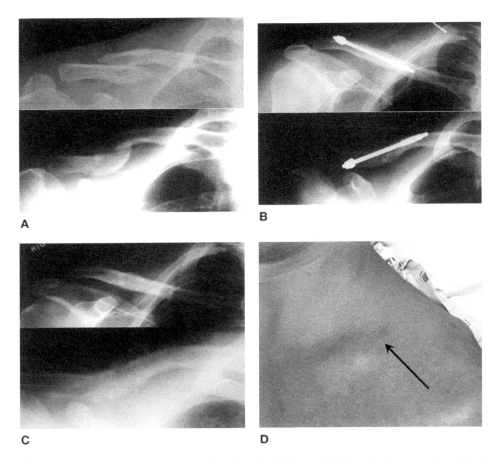

A

B

C

D

Figure 20 Radiographs of a malunion showing injury, malunion, pin placement, and final result.

fracture site can be demonstrated by performing a cross-body adduction view of the shoulder (Fig. 21). This stress x-ray will accentuate conoid ligament detachment from the medial clavicular fragment. Positive findings include an increase in fracture displacement, an increase in the CC interval, and marked underriding of the distal fragment beneath the proximal fragment. This is medial rotational instability occurring through the fracture site. Failure of this to occur suggests the conoid ligament is still attached to the medial fragment of the clavicle. A good MRI scan will also demonstrate the CC ligaments.

For the unstable variety of this fracture, we generally prefer placement of a coracoclavicular screw, which will reduce the coracoclavicular interval and therefore bring the fragments into close proximity to allow healing. Other options include plate fixation, coracoclavicular suture circlage, and some advocate K-wire fixation. Plate fixation of this fracture can be problematic. The required exposure is relatively large. The distal fragment is small, and the AC joint limits the length of plate that can be used. A small T-plate sometimes allows enough screws in the distal fragment

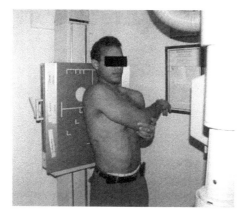

Figure 21   Positioning to obtain a cross-body adduction AP of the shoulder.

for adequate fixation. K-wire fixation down the intramedullary canal of the distal clavicle can create problems as well. The forces on this area are large, and hardware failure is quite possible. Migration of broken hardware in this region is well documented, and we recommend avoidance of this technique.

The CC screw offers several advantages. The required exposure is small, and the fracture site does not necessarily require open exposure. The fixation is solid, and using C-arm guidance this procedure can be performed almost percutaneously. After fracture healing, the screw can be removed easily under local anesthesia, thereby avoiding breakage of the hardware.

VII   TECHNIQUE FOR CORACOCLAVICULAR SCREW FIXATION

The beach chair position using a radiolucent positioner is required to obtain the necessary medial oblique view of the coracoid and clavicle. The C-arm is positioned prior to patient prep to confirm that the appropriate view is obtainable. The base of the machine is positioned at the head of the table, with the C-arm "over the top" of the shoulder similar to the technique used in midshaft fractures. The one important variation is that the receiver is placed as far medial as the bed will allow. The beam is directed from anterolateral to posteromedial. The view of the coracoid thus obtained must be "down the barrel" of the coracoid, which produces a nearly perfect dense circle (Fig. 22). The circle or "target" is the x-ray shadow of the combined cortical density of the shaft of the coracoid with the intramedullary cancellous bone as the clear central region of the target. This target view with a nearly perfect circle must be obtained prior to proceeding. If it cannot be obtained, you must readjust the C-arm and/or the table to get this view. More often than not, the base of the receiver is not far enough medial. This view will allow you to place the CC screw in perfect position every time. Improper positioning of the C-arm risks malposition of the screw and fixation failure.

The shoulder and upper extremity are prepped in standard fashion with the upper extremity draped free to allow full motion if necessary. The site for the skin incision is located using C-arm guidance. The appropriate position is overlying the

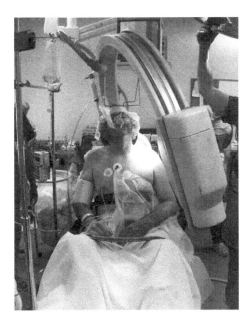

Figure 22 Positioning of the C-arm for coracoclavicular fixation of the AC joint. The C-arm should be oriented in a posteromedial to anterolateral manner to get the beam parallel to the coracoid.

clavicle just medial to the conoid tubercle on the inferior surface of the clavicle. The incision extends from the posterior border of the clavicle to the anterior border of the clavicle. The anterior and posterior borders of the clavicle are identified using subperiosteal dissection. We prefer to use the Rockwood screw set (Depuy). The 3/16″ (large) drill bit is centered on the dorsal surface of the medial fragment of the clavicle just medial to the conoid tubercle. The drill tip is aimed toward the base of the coracoid, which usually requires the drill hand to be up against the ipsilateral side of the patient's head. Both cortices of the clavicle are drilled, and the hole is then widened by toggling the drill in the hole. This allows some latitude with the small (9/64″) drill bit to allow placement in the exact center of the coracoid base. The 9/64″ (small) drill bit is then passed through the clavicular drill hole and is used to "palpate" the base of the coracoid. The tip of the drill bit is used to locate the medial and lateral borders of the coracoid. These positions are confirmed on the C-arm. The drill bit is then positioned at the top of the target circle so as to pierce the center of the target from superior to inferior. With the fracture held in a reduced position, the first cortex is drilled. This is usually relatively weak bone. The intramedullary bone provides no resistance to the drill. The inferior cortex is solid bone and provides good tactile and auditory feedback at the point of penetration. Drill penetration of the inferior cortex is confirmed on C-arm. A depth gauge is used to measure the appropriate length screw and to confirm the angle of screw placement. Usually a 45 or 50 mm screw with a washer is appropriate for the average sized male. The screw is passed through the clavicle, and then the screw tip should be placed at the top of the target to allow the nipple of the screw to seat in the drill hole. This is felt and

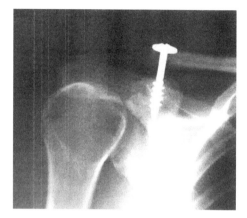

Figure 23 Final placement of the coracoclavicular screw in the center of the coracoid base.

confirmed using the C-arm intensifier. The screw is then tightened into position piercing the center of the target under C-arm guidance. The inferior cortex must be engaged to obtain solid fixation (Fig. 23). We have successfully used this same procedure for nonunions of distal clavicle fractures. Since the fracture occurs in a more cancellous portion of the clavicle, good healing can usually be obtained once the nonunion site is curetted and bone grafted.

Postoperatively the patient is placed into a sling and swathe with later transition to a sling for comfort only. The patient is allowed to perform activities of daily living with the extremity and to lift up to 5 pounds. The patient is told not to use his or her arm with the hands higher than the shoulder. When the fracture shows radiographic healing, the screw is removed, generally under local anesthesia.

BIBLIOGRAPHY

Abbot LC, and Lucas DB: Function of the clavicle. Its surgical significance. Ann Surg 1954; 140:583–599.

Anderson K, Jensen P, Lauritzen J. Treatment of clavicular fractures. Figure of eight bandage vs a simple sling. Acta Orthop Scand 1987; 57:71–74.

Berkheiser EJ. Old ununited clavicular fractures in the adult. Surg Gynecol Obstet 1937; 64:1064–1072.

Breck L. Partially threaded round pins with oversized threads for intramedullary fixation of the clavicle and the forearm bones. Clin Orthop 1958; 11:227–229.

Campbell E, Howard WB, Breklund CW. Delayed brachial plexus palsy due to ununited fracture of the clavicle. JAMA 1949; 139:91–92.

Depalma A. Surgery of the Shoulder. 3rd ed. Philadelphia: JB Lippincott, 1983.

Dugdale TW, Fulkerson JB: Pneumothorax complicating a closed fracture of the clavicle. A case report. Clin Orthop 1987; 221:212–214.

Edvardsen P, Odegard O: Treatment of posttraumatic clavicular pseudoarthrosis. Acta Orthop Scand 1977; 48:456–457.

Grazier KL, Holbrook TL, Kelsey JL, Stauffer RN. The Frequency of Occurrence, Impact, and Cost of Musculoskeletal Conditions in the United States. American Academy of Orthopaedic Surgeons, 1984.

Howard FM, and Schafer SJ. Injuries to the clavicle with neurovascular complications. A study of fourteen cases. JBJS 1965; 47A:1335–1346.

Hoyer HE, Kindt R, Lippert H. Zur Biomechanik der menschlichen Clavicula. Z Orthop 1980; 118:915–922.

Inman VT, Saunders JB: Observation in the function of the clavicle. Clin Med 1946; 65:158–165.

Jablon M, Sutker A, Post M. Irreducible fractures of the middle third of the clavicle. JBJS 1979; 61A:296–298.

Javid H. Vascular Injuries of the neck. Clin Orthop 1963; 28:70–78.

Jit I, Kulkrani M. Times of appearance and fusion of epiphysis at the medial end of the clavicle. Ind J Med Res 1976; 64(5):773–792.

Jupiter JB, Leffert RD. Nonunion of the clavicle. JBJS 1987; 69A:753–760.

Khan MAA, Lucas HK. Plating of fractures of the middle third of the clavicle. Injury 1978; 9:263–267.

Kay SP, Eckardt JJ. Brachial plexus palsy secondary to clavicular nonunion. A case report and interature survey. Clin Orthop 1986; 206:219–222.

Klier I, Mayor PB. Laceration of the innominate internal jugular venous junction. Rare complication of fracture of the clavicle. Orthop Rev 1981; 10:81–82.

Lengua F, Nuss JM, Lechner R, Baruthio J, Veillon F. [The treatment of fracture of the clavicle by closed medio lateral pinning.] Rev Chir Orthop 1987; 73(5):377–380.

Lim E, Day LJ. Subclavian vein thrombosis following fracture of the clavicle. A case report. Orthopedics 1987; 10(2):349–351.

Ljunggren AE. Clavicular function. Acta Orthop Scand 1979; 50:261–268.

Luskin R, Weiss CA, Winer J. The role of the sublavius muscle in the subclavian vein syndrome (costoclavicular syndrome) following fracture of the clavicle. Clin Orthop 1967; 54:75–84.

Manske DJ, Szabo RM. The operative treatment of mid-shaft clavicular non-unions. JBJS 1985; 67A:1367–1371.

Matry C. Fracture de la clavicule gauche au tiers interne. Blessure de la vein sour-claviere. Osteosynthese Bull Mem Soc Nat Chir 1932; 58:75–78.

McCandless DN, Mowbray M. Treatment of displaced fractures of the clavicle. Sling vs figure of eight bandage. Practitioner 1979; 223:266–267.

Moore TO. Internal pin fixation for fracture of the clavicle. Am Surg 1951; 17:580–583.

Moseley HF. In: Shoulder Lesions. Edinburgh: Churchill Livingstone, 1972:207–235.

Mueller ME, Allgower N, Willenegger H. Manual of Internal Fixation. New York: Springer-Verlag, 1970.

Murray G. A method of fixation for fracture of the clavicle. J Bone Joint Surg 1940; 22:616–620.

Neviaser RJ, Neviaser JS, Neviaser TJ. A simple technique for internal fixation of the clavicle. Clin Orthop 1975; 109:103–107.

Neer CS II. Fractures of the clavicle. In: Rockwood CA, Green DP, eds. Fractures in Adults. Philadelphia: JB Lippincott, 1984:707–713.

Ogden JA, Conologue GJ, Bronson NL. Radiology of postnatal skeletal development. Vol. 3. The clavicle. Skel Radiol 1979; 4:196–203.

Paffen PJ, Jansen EW. Surgical treatment of clavicular fractures with Kirshner wires. A comparative study. Arch Chir Neerl 1978; 30:43–53.

Perry B. An improved clavicular pin. Am J Surg 1966; 112:142–144.

Rockwood CA. Personal communications, 1993–1997.

Rowe CR. An atlas of anatomy and treatment of mid-clavicular fractures. Clin Orthop 1968; 58:29–42.

Rush LV, Rush HL. Technique of longitudinal pin fixation in fractures of the clavicle and jaw. Mississippi Doctor 1949; 27:332.

Sakellarides H. Pseudoarthrosis of the clavicle. JBJS 1961; 43A:130–138.

Sankarankutty M, Turner BW: Fractures of the clavicle. Injury 1975; 7(2):101–106.

Silloway KA, Mclaughlin RE, Edlichy RC, et al. Clavicular fractures and acromioclavicular joint injures in lacrosse: preventable injuries. J Emerg Med 1985; 3:117–121.

Spar I. Total clavulectomy for pathologic fractures. Clin Orthop 1977; 129:236–237.

Stanley D, Trowbridge EA, Norris SH. The mechanism of clavicular fracture. JBJS 1988; 70B:461–464.

Tse DH, Slabaugh PB, Carlson PA. Injury to the axillary artery by a closed fracture of the clavicle. JBJS 1980; 62A:1372–1373.

Tyrnin AH. The Bohler clavicle splint in the treatment of clavicular injuries. J Bone Joint Surg 1937; 19:417–424.

Zenni EJ, Krieg JK, Rosen MJ. Open reduction and internal fixation of clavicular fractures. J Bone Joint Surg 1981; 63-A:147–151.

Eskola A, Vainionpaa S, Myllynen P, Patiala H, Rokkanen P. Outcome of clavicular fracture in 89 patients. Arch Orthop Trauma Surg 1986; 105:337–338.

Hill JM, McGuire MH, Crosby LA. Closed treatment of displaced middle-third fractures of the clavicle gives poor results. J Bone Joint Surg 1997; 79-B:537–539.

Basamania CJ. "Claviculoplasty" and intramedullary fixation of malunited clavicle fractures. Presented at International Congress of Shoulder Surgery, Syndney, Australia, 1999.

Ballmer FT, Gerber C. Coracoclavicular screw fixation for unstable fractures of the distal clavicle. A report of five cases. J Bone Joint Surg 1991; 73-B:291–294.

14

Humeral Shaft Fractures: Surgical Approaches

GREGORY S. BAUER

Goldsboro Orthopaedic Associates, Goldsboro, North Carolina, U.S.A.

THEODORE A. BLAINE

Columbia University, College of Physicians and Surgeons, New York-Presbyterian Hospital, and Center for Shoulder, Elbow and Sports Medicine, New York, New York, U.S.A.

I INTRODUCTION

Humeral shaft fractures are classified according to location, extent of comminution, presence or absence of intra-articular extension, and associated injuries. When simple extra-articular fractures of the humeral shaft are present without associated injuries, nonoperative treatment is appropriate. However, when surgical treatment of humeral shaft fractures is required, there are many pearls and pitfalls that are important to review. The present chapter will focus on the surgical approaches to the humeral shaft and outline the authors' preferences for the treatment of various fractures.

II PREOPERATIVE PLANNING

Preoperative planning, as in all fractures, is a critical component of treatment in humeral shaft fractures. Radiographs must be obtained in two planes. For more proximal fractures, an axillary view may also be helpful; while in more distal fractures, anteroposterior (AP), lateral, and oblique views of the elbow should also be obtained. The type of fracture and fracture configuration will dictate much of the preoperative planning. If extensive comminution is present, it may be necessary to obtain contralateral views in order to assess arm length. When intramedullary (IM) nailing is considered, intraoperative fluoroscopy or plain radiography may be necessary and should be arranged in advance. Finally, all potential implants should be available at surgery, including various plates, screws, bone reduction forceps, and any other implants of choice. In operative reduction of fractures of the humeral shaft, exposure of neurovascular structures is often required and loupe magnification is recommended.

III SURGICAL TREATMENT

The entire arm including the shoulder should be prepped in all cases to allow for extension of the surgical exposure if required. When extensive comminution is present or surgery is planned for fracture nonunion, the hip should be prepared and draped in anticipation of a possible bone graft. There are several operative approaches available depending upon the fracture location, associated injuries, and surgeon's preference. The authors' preference for each fracture type is listed in Table 1, and each approach is presented here in detail.

IV SURGICAL APPROACHES

A Anterior Approach

The anterior approach to the humerus is an extension of the deltopectoral incision and provides exposure from the glenohumeral joint proximally to the coronoid fossa distally (1). It is useful for the treatment of fractures of the proximal two thirds of the humerus and is the recommended approach for fractures involving the proximal one third of the humerus. A plate applied for osteosynthesis will fit nicely on either the anterior or lateral surface of the proximal two thirds of the humeral diaphysis.

Proximally, the surgical interval is between the deltoid (axillary nerve) and the pectoralis major (medial and lateral pectoral nerves). Distally, the interval is between the lateral and medial fibers of the brachialis supplied by the radial and musculocutaneous nerves, respectively.

The patient is positioned in either a modified beach chair or supine position. The coracoid process is palpated, and the intended incision is drawn from just lateral to the tip of the coracoid toward the deltoid insertion in the deltopectoral groove. The incision can extend to the flexion crease distally as it gently curves to follow the biceps tendon (Fig. 1). The entire exposure is rarely required for fracture fixation. The interval between the pectoralis major and the deltoid is developed proximally. The key to this interval is the cephalic vein that runs in the interval and is often

Table 1 Preferred Surgical Approaches

Fracture location	Surgical approach
Proximal 1/3	Anterior
Middle 1/3	Anterolateral or posterior
Distal 1/3	Posterior
Nonunion	Posterior

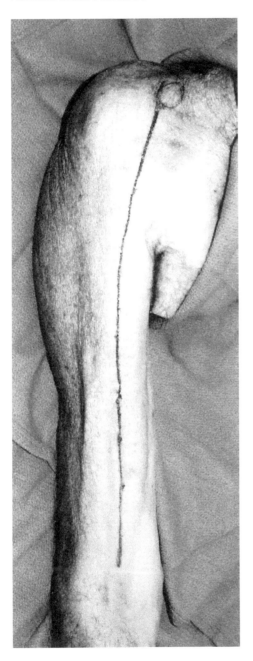

Figure 1   The skin incision for the anterior approach is carried from the coracoid process proximally, over the deltopectoral groove and continues with a gentle curve following the lateral edge of the biceps to the flexion crease of the elbow.

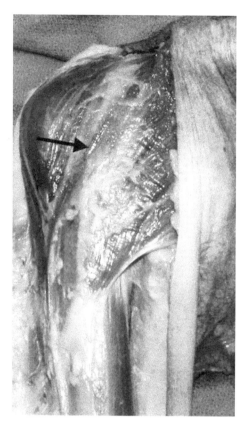

Figure 2 The key landmark proximally is the cephalic vein (black arrow) that marks the deltopectoral interval.

surrounded by a stripe of fat (Fig. 2). The vein can be taken either medially or laterally, but receives more branches from the deltoid, thus less bleeding is encountered if it stays with the deltoid laterally. Once the vein is protected, the interval is developed proximally where a triangle is formed between the clavicular head of the pectoralis major and the anterior deltoid.

The clavipectoral fascia is then incised and a retractor is placed under the conjoined tendon of the coracobrachialis and the short head of the biceps. Adhesions under the deltoid should be released from the deltoid insertion up to the acromion. The axillary nerve, which courses around the posterior humerus 3–8 cm distal to the acromion, must be palpated and preserved during subdeltoid dissection. There are often adhesions from the deltoid to the coracoacromial ligament that should be released, further facilitating exposure. A retractor is then placed under the deltoid with care taken to avoid excess force. The periosteum is incised lateral to the insertion of the pectoralis major tendon. If necessary for further exposure, a portion of the pectoralis major tendon can be released lateral to the bicipital groove. The tendon should be tagged with a nonabsorbable suture to facilitate mobilization and reattachment at the end of the procedure. Care is taken to avoid injuring the tendon of the long head of the biceps. The ascending branch of the anterior humeral circumflex vessel will be encountered at the lateral edge of the bicipital groove. A portion of the deltoid insertion can be released if necessary for exposure; however, this is not routinely recommended.

Further proximal exposure requires takedown of the subscapularis tendon. The tendon is released 1 cm medial to its insertion on the lesser tuberosity, leaving a healthy cuff of tissue for reapproximation. The anterior humeral circumflex artery and its two accompanying veins run along the inferior border of the tendinous portion of the subscapularis and will require ligation or cauterization (arrow, Fig. 3). The axillary nerve runs with the posterior humeral circumflex artery under the muscular portion of the subscapularis on its way to the quadrilateral space and must be protected.

Distally, once the skin is incised, the deep fascia is incised over the interval between the biceps and the brachialis. Care is taken to continue to protect the cephalic vein. The mobile biceps is retracted medially further exposing the brachialis. In the distal portion of the wound, the lateral antebrachial cutaneous nerve is found in the interval between the brachialis and biceps, just lateral to the biceps tendon at the level of the epicondylar line (2) (arrow, Fig. 4). This should be identified and preserved. The brachialis is then split longitudinally in the midline, and this can extend to its tendinous insertion on the coronoid process of the ulna (Fig. 5). Flexing

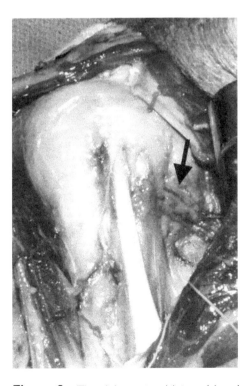

Figure 3 The deltopectoral interval has been developed with the pectoralis major and conjoined tendon retracted medially and the deltoid laterally with the cephalic vein. Note the anterior humeral circumflex vessels (black arrow) traversing the subscapularis.

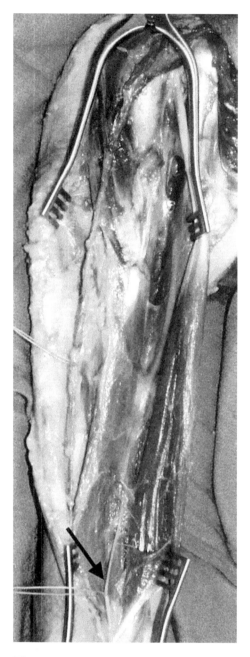

Figure 4 The biceps has been retracted medially exposing the brachialis. The lateral antebrachial cutaneous nerve is found in this interval just lateral to the distal biceps tendon at the level of the epicondylar line (black arrow).

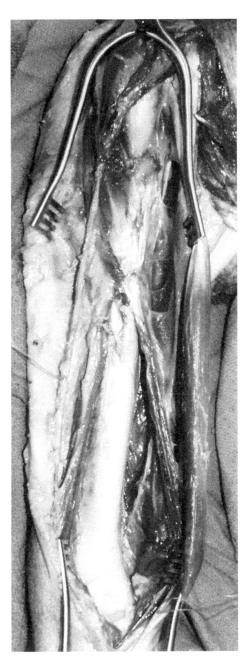

Figure 5 The brachialis fibers and periosteum have been split longitudinally, exposing the humerus to the level of the coronoid fossa.

the elbow will decrease the tension on the brachialis, facilitating distal exposure allowing visualization of the trochlea and coronoid fossa. Laterally, the radial nerve, which pierces the lateral intermuscular septum 10 cm proximal to the lateral epicondyle to enter the anterior compartment of the arm, should be protected (3). The periosteum is split longitudinally. The soft tissues should be elevated subperiosteally to avoid injury to the radial nerve laterally and the ulnar nerve medially, which runs just posterior to the medial intermuscular septum.

B   Anterolateral Approach to the Humerus

This approach provides exposure to the distal half of the humerus and is especially useful for fractures involving this region with neurological compromise of the radial nerve. It allows direct visualization and exploration of the radial nerve. It can also be extended distally as an anterior approach to the elbow between the brachioradialis and the pronator teres (4).

The surgical interval superficially is between the biceps (musculocutaneous), which is retracted medially from the brachialis (musculocutaneous medially and radial nerve laterally). The deep interval involves muscles all innervated by the radial nerve. The lateral fibers of the brachialis are elevated medially while the brachioradialis and lateral head of the triceps is elevated laterally.

The patient is positioned supine or in the modified beach chair position. The skin incision follows the lateral border of the biceps muscle, proximally from the pectoralis tendon to the elbow flexion crease distally (Fig. 6). The fascia is incised in line with the skin incision with care taken to preserve the cephalic vein. The biceps is retracted medially exposing the brachialis underneath. The lateral antebrachial cutaneous nerve is found in this interval just lateral to the biceps tendon at the level of the epicondylar line (Fig. 7) (2). This should be identified and preserved, retracting it medially with the biceps. In order to expose the radial nerve, the interval between the brachialis medially and the brachioradialis laterally is developed (Fig. 8). After the fascia is incised, the interval is carefully explored distally. Finding the nerve is critical to this exposure. It is helpful to gently palpate for the nerve.

Once the nerve is identified in the interval distally, it can be traced proximal to the lateral intermuscular septum, where it enters the anterior compartment from the posterior compartment through the lateral intermuscular septum 10 cm proximal to the lateral epicondyle (3). The radial nerve and the brachioradialis are retracted laterally. The radial nerve is extremely sensitive to manipulation and should be carefully isolated with a vessel loop (Fig. 9). The periosteum is sharply incised at the lateral border of the brachialis and the muscle subperiosteally elevated exposing the humerus (Fig. 10). Distally, exposure can be extended by developing the interval between the brachioradialis laterally and the pronator teres (median nerve) medially as an anterior approach to the elbow. Proximally, continue the subperiosteal elevation of the brachialis, which is separated from the lateral head of the triceps by the lateral intermuscular septum. All posterior dissection must be performed subperiosteally to prevent injury to the radial nerve as it passes through the spiral groove on its way to the lateral intermuscular septum.

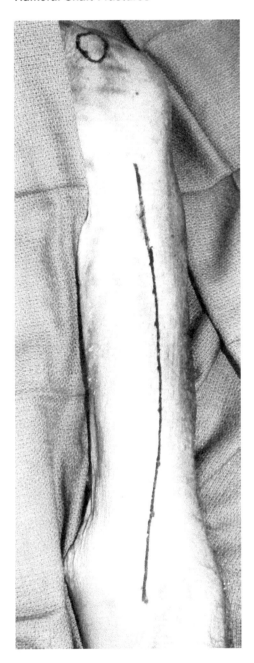

Figure 6 The skin incision for the anterolateral approach is made just lateral to the biceps from the pectoralis tendon proximally to the elbow flexion crease distally.

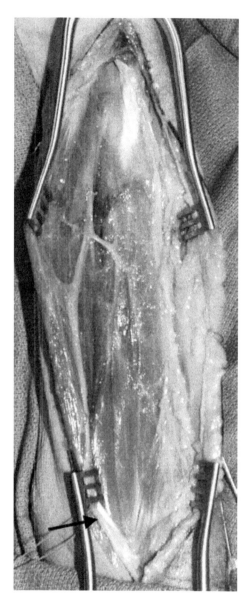

Figure 7 The biceps has been retracted medially to expose the brachialis. The lateral antebrachial cutaneous nerve is protected medially (black arrow).

C Medial Approach to the Humerus

The medial approach to the humerus provides exposure to the middle third of the humerus. It is rarely used due to the potential damage to the neurovascular structures. Its use is indicated when soft tissue damage to other parts of the humerus prevents the use of another approach (5). The interval is developed between the

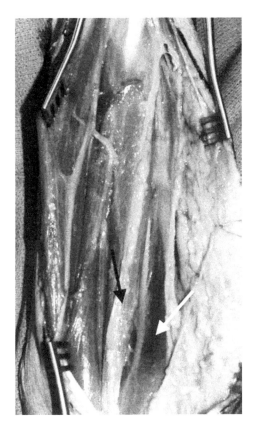

Figure 8 The interval between the brachialis medially (black arrow) and the brachioradialis laterally (white arrow) is developed.

flexor compartment anteriorly (musculocutaneous nerve) and the long head of the triceps (radial nerve) posteriorly.

The patient is positioned supine with the arm abducted 90° and placed on an arm board. The skin incision is along the bicipital sulcus from the axillary fold to the medial epicondyle (Fig. 11) (6). The subcutaneous tissue is divided. The cutaneous nerves that run in the adipose tissue are protected by developing full-thickness flaps. The fascia is divided anterior to the medial intermuscular septum. The median nerve is isolated with the brachial artery anteriorly. There are several crossing vessels to the brachial vessels that will require ligation or cauterization to facilitate mobilization anteriorly. The ulnar nerve, along with the accompanying superior ulnar collateral artery and vein, passes through the septum from anterior to posterior 8 cm proximal to the medial epicondyle and is identified and preserved (Fig. 12) (7). Once the neurovascular structures are safely protected, the periosteum is split longitudinally just in front of the medial intermuscular septum between the brachialis and coracobrachialis anteriorly and the long head of the triceps posteriorly (Fig. 13). These muscles are then elevated subperiosteally anteriorly and posteriorly, respectively, exposing the humerus (Fig. 14).

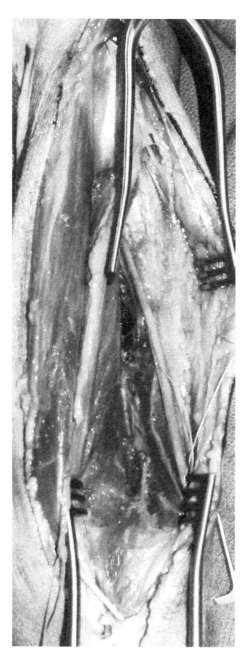

Figure 9 The radial nerve is isolated and retracted laterally with the brachioradialis.

D Posterior Approach to the Humerus

The posterior approach provides exposure to the distal two thirds of the humerus. It is used for diaphyseal fractures in the distal half of the humerus where the posterior surface is relatively flat and accepts a plate for osteosynthesis. Midshaft fractures

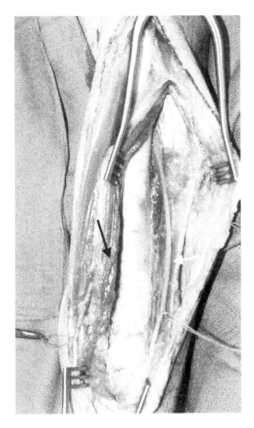

Figure 10 The lateral border of the brachialis is subperiosteally elevated medially (black arrow) while the brachioradialis (white arrow) is elevated laterally exposing the humerus.

with neurological injury of the radial nerve that require open reduction and internal fixation should be approached posteriorly, as the posterior approach provides for exploration of the radial nerve as it courses along the spiral groove. For more distal fractures, care should be taken to ensure that the plate does not enter the olecranon fossa preventing full extension of the elbow. There is no true internervous plane as the interval involves splitting the heads of the triceps muscle, which are all innervated by branches of the radial nerve. Superficially, the long head is split from the lateral head while the deep dissection involves longitudinally splitting the fibers of the medial head.

The patient is positioned either in the lateral decubitus position with the arm abducted 90° or prone with the arm either abducted or adducted. The acromion is palpated as well as the olecranon process and the mobile long head of the triceps. The incision begins three fingerbreadths below the posterior edge of the acromion along the lateral edge of the long head of the triceps to the tip of the olecranon (Fig. 15) (1). The proximal extent of exposure is limited by the posterior deltoid. Once appropriate skin flaps have been developed, the fascia is opened proximally between the long and lateral heads of the triceps (Fig. 16). These muscles can safely be split as

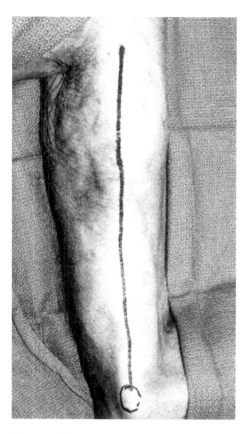

Figure 11   The skin incision for the medial approach is along the bicipital sulcus from the axillary fold to the medial epicondyle.

they receive their innervation quite proximally, 7.1 cm and 10.1 cm from the tip of the acromion, respectively (8).

This muscular interval can be developed bluntly with the use of a soft tissue elevator dividing the fibers of the long head medially from the lateral head fibers laterally until the appearance of the common tendon distally. Once the radial nerve is identified and preserved, the tendinous portion of the triceps is sharply divided from proximal to distal (Fig. 17). Beneath the superficial layer of the long and lateral heads is the deep medial head of the triceps. The radial nerve and profuda brachii artery, which travel from proximal medial to distal lateral, lie in the spiral groove that runs along the superior lateral border of the medial head, separating it from the lateral head.

Once the radial nerve is located it can be isolated along with the profuda brachii artery using a vessel loop (Fig. 18). The medial head of the triceps can now be

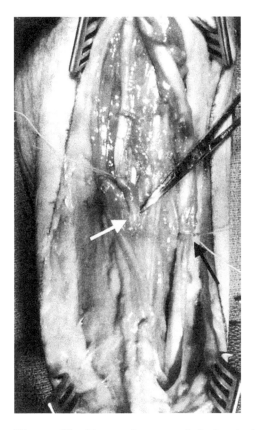

Figure 12 The median nerve is isolated with the brachial artery (black arrow) and the ulnar with the superior ulnar collateral artery. It is seen entering the posterior compartment through the medial intermuscular septum (white arrow).

split midline down to bone as the fibers have separate innervation. The ulnar collateral branch of the radial nerve, which runs closely with the ulnar nerve, innervates the medial fibers, and the lateral fibers receive branches from the posterior muscular branch, which also supplies the lateral head and the anconeus (8). All dissection should continue subperiosteally to avoid injury to the ulnar nerve medially that passes from the anterior to the posterior compartment of the arm through the medial intermuscular septum 8 cm proximal to the medial epicondyle (7). Flexing the elbow will expose the olecranon fossa. A meticulous repair of the tendon is performed preventing postoperative disruption of the extensor mechanism.

V TECHNIQUES OF FIXATION

A Plates

Plate fixation of humeral shaft fractures is performed with attention to AO principles. Interfragmentary lag screws should be used whenever possible. Compression should be achieved across the fracture site and every effort should

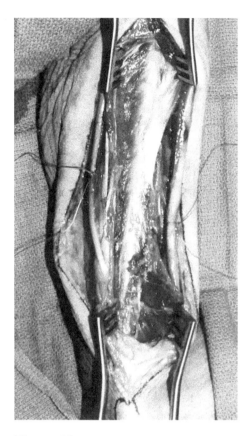

Figure 13 The neurovascular structures have been protected and retracted anteriorly and posteriorly. The periosteum is exposed.

be made to obtain eight cortices proximal and distal to the fracture site. Occasionally, six cortices may be accepted when there is no fracture comminution and interfragmentary compression is achieved. The 4.5 broad dynamic compression plate (DCP) (AO Research Institute, Davos, Switzerland) is an excellent choice for plate application on the posterior humerus while the thinner 4.5 low contact LC-DCP (AO Research Institute) may be required for anterior or anterolateral plate application. 4.5 DCP plates are also an excellent choice for fixation of distal humerus fractures along the columns (Figs. 19, 20) Plates should always be used in the setting of fracture nonunion as IM nails have virtually no role in this setting. The addition of autogenous bone graft is required in the setting of atrophic nonunions and may also be necessary in cases of extensive comminution.

   Plate fixation of humeral shaft fractures has had consistently successful results. Several series have reported on the excellent results of plate fixation for acute humeral shaft fractures, with union rates from 97 to 100% (9–14). Plate fixation has also been used successfully in the presence of fracture nonunion, with union rates ranging from 80 to 100% (15). Plate fixation is currently the gold standard for treatment of factures of the humeral shaft not amenable to closed treatment.

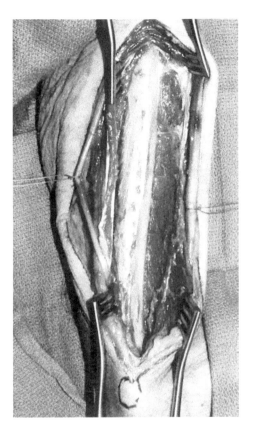

Figure 14 The brachialis and coroacobrachialis are subperiosteally elevated anteriorly while the long head of the triceps is elevated posteriorly exposing the humerus.

B Intramedullary Fixation

Intramedullary fixation of humeral shaft fractures has had a recent resurgence in interest. Its indications include multiple trauma, segmental fracture or floating shoulder/elbow, or inability to control the fracture by closed treatment. Rush rods and enders nails have been used for fractures of the proximal humerus with some success. However, they provide inadequate fracture stability and should not be considered for fractures of the humeral shaft.

Locked intramedullary nails may be used with either antegrade or retrograde insertion. Retrograde nail insertion has been advocated to avoid the high incidence of rotator cuff problems with antegrade nail insertion. Retrograde nail insertion may be technically difficult, however, and care should be taken not to violate the supracondylar columns during nail insertion, which may lead to iatrogenic fracture. Important principles in intramedullary nailing include avoidance of distraction at the fracture site, the routine use of proximal and distal locking screws inserted under direct vision to avoid neural injury.

The results of intramedullary nailing of humeral shaft fractures approaches the results of plate fixation, with union rates of 86–100% in various series (13,14).

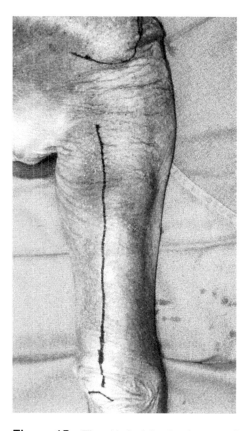

Figure 15 The skin incision for the posterior approach begins three fingerbreadths below the posterior edge of the acromion along the lateral edge of the long head of the triceps to the olecranon tip.

However, shoulder pain and impingement are a consistent phenomenon, occasionally requiring an additional operation for nail removal (16,17). These findings have led other authors to recommend retrograde nail insertion to avoid violation of the rotator cuff. Two recent series have reported excellent results with this technique, with no incidence of shoulder dysfunction and little incidence of elbow stiffness (18–20).

C External Fixation

There are few indications for external fixation of the humeral shaft. Rare indications include multiple trauma requiring immediate stable fixation, soft tissue compromise, infection, and fracture nonunion. Various types of external fixation devices are available and include frame constructs composed of threaded half-pins, thin-wire ring fixators, hybrid frame constructs (Fig. 21), as well as articulated frames. A comprehensive knowledge of the regional anatomy is important to avoid potential neurovascular injury. For placement of lateral pins in the distal humerus, an open approach is recommended to avoid injury to the radial nerve. When pins are required for more proximal and distal fractures, pins should be placed in an extrarticular location to avoid joint sepsis.

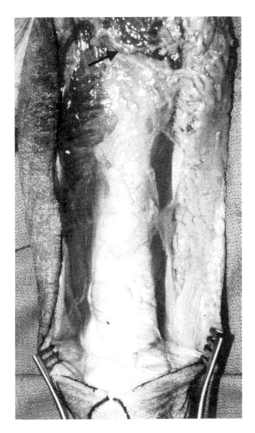

Figure 16   Flaps are developed to facilitate exposure. The deltoid (arrow) limits exposure proximally.

The results of external fixation for humeral shaft fractures have been variable based upon the presenting pathology and the surgical technique. Because of the rarity of acute humeral shaft fractures treated with primary external fixation, only a few series have reported these results; however, the results from these series have been excellent, with union rates of 95–98% (21,22). External fixation of the humeral shaft is more commonly used in the setting of complicated and open humeral shaft fractures, and these results have been less successful. Three series in which a small wire ring fixator were used for humerus fracture nonunions reported successful union in 80–93% of cases, and the average time to healing ranged from 4.5 to 7.5 months in these series (23–25).

VI   AUTHORS' PREFERENCES

A   Surgical Approach

The most commonly used surgical approaches to the humeral shaft are the anterolateral and posterior approaches, and decision as to which to use has been largely based on surgeon preference (see Table 1). Because of the potential risk of

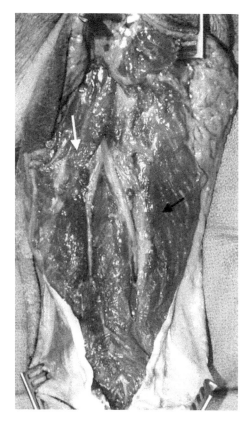

Figure 17 The long (white arrow) and lateral (black arrow) heads have been split exposing the medial head with the radial nerve on its superior border.

injury to the radial nerve, the posterior approach is our preferred approach for all primary fractures of the humeral shaft except those involving the proximal one third. For nonunions, scarring around the fracture site makes exposure of all neurovascular structures imperative, and therefore the posterior approach is also preferred.

B Preferred Operative Technique

While intramedullary fixation has been proven to provide excellent results in some series, the increased incidence of shoulder dysfunction with antegrade nail insertion, as well as a higher nonunion rate, makes this technique less desirable. Retrograde nail insertion is preferred when IM nailing is performed. However, given the high success rate of open plating techniques, we prefer open reduction and internal fixation for all acute fractures of the humeral shaft, which require surgery.

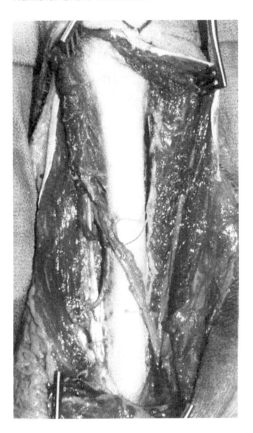

Figure 18 The fibers of the medial head are split midline exposing the humerus while the radial nerve and accompanying profunda brachii artery have been isolated and protected.

VII PEARLS AND PITFALLS

A Neurological Injury

Due to the close proximity of the radial nerve to the humeral shaft in the spiral groove, neurological injury is unfortunately a major concern with internal fixation of humeral shaft fractures. Postoperative radial nerve injury has been reported in 1–10% of patients. Injury can occur indirectly during IM nailing if the reamer is left on while crossing the fracture site. It is therefore imperative that the reamer be stopped while traversing the fracture site and restarted when distal. This necessitates that reaming of humeral shaft fracture be performed under fluoroscopic image. For plate fixation of humeral shaft fractures, we recommend direct exposure and protection of the radial nerve, and this is best performed with the posterior approach. In revision cases or cases of nonunion, it is often necessary to extend the incision to locate the nerve either proximally or distally to prevent neurologic injury. In distal one third fractures, the posterior approach is always used and the ulnar nerve must be isolated, exposed, and typically transposed at the conclusion of the procedure.

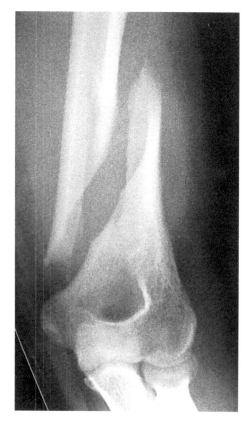

Figure 19 Preoperative anteroposterior radiograph showing a displaced spiral distal humerus fracture in an obese patient.

B Nonunions

Nonunion of fractures of the humeral shaft occur rarely, but may be associated with open fractures, infection, or failed internal fixation due to either patient factors or surgical factors. Union of a humeral shaft fracture typically occurs in 8–12 weeks, and a delay in this process is indicative of delayed union. When all potential for fracture healing has been lost, usually by 4–6 months in the humeral shaft, a nonunion is present. Nonunions of humeral shaft fractures can be very difficult to treat, and therefore, all efforts to avoid potential nonunion should be made during initial fracture treatment. These considerations include:

1. Preoperative factors, including adequate patient selection and avoidance of internal fixation in patients with premorbidities and potential risk of infection.
2. Surgical factors, including avoidance of devascularizing the fracture fragments by excessive stripping and attention to sufficient fracture fixation with plates of adequate length. Bone graft should be added to those fractures with excessive comminution.

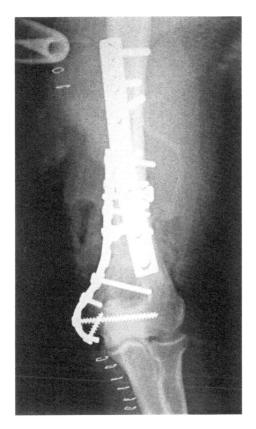

Figure 20 Postoperative anteroposterior radiograph showing fixation of spiral distal humerus fracture with a posteriorly applied 4.5 DCP plate and a medial 3.5 pelvic reconstruction plate.

3. Avoidance of intramedullary nails in most cases.
4. Postoperative considerations, including appropriate rehabilitation while avoiding overaggressive therapy that may place fixation at risk.

With attention to these details, nonunion of humeral shaft fractures can be avoided in the majority of cases. When nonunion is present, potential treatment options include open reduction and internal fixation or external fixation (26,27). There is no role for intramedullary nailing of humeral shaft nonunions (28). In the presence of an infected nonunion, external fixation may be considered (25) (Figs. 21, 22) Results using this technique have led to successful results in up to 80% of patients. When infection is not present, internal fixation with plate and iliac crest bone graft is the treatment of choice (15). In rare cases of atrophic nonunion with severe bone loss, vascularized fibular grafting may be required (29). With these techniques utilizing either iliac crest or fibular grafting, union rates of 93% have been reported.

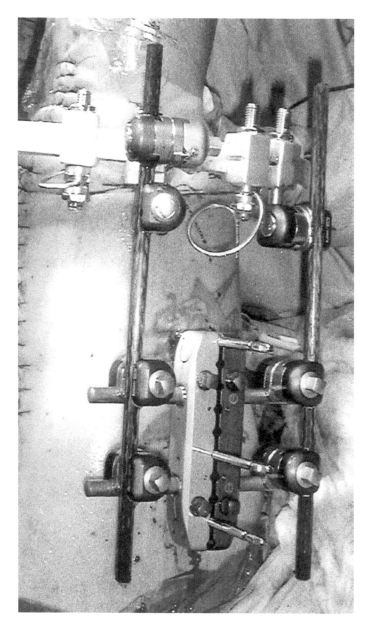

Figure 21 Intraoperative photograph following application of a hybrid external fixation frame for an infected distal humerus nonunion.

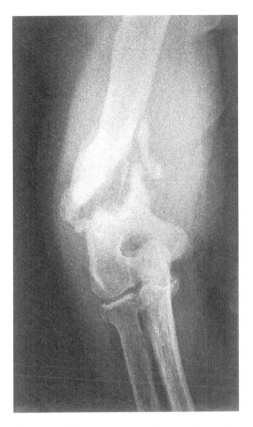

Figure 22 Anteroposterior radiograph demonstrating an infected distal humerus nonunion.

VIII POSTOPERATIVE REHABILITATION

Early mobilization is the primary goal of achieving stable internal fixation of proximal humerus fractures. Thus, mobilization should be commenced as soon as fracture stability is ensured and wound healing is satisfactory. If the fracture is stably internally fixed, we will begin gentle passive and active assistive range of motion in the first 7–10 days postoperatively. Emphasis is placed upon shoulder and elbow range of motion. Attention also should be directed at hand and finger mobilization, which can be compromised by excessive swelling and may lead to the shoulder-hand syndrome, a form of reflex sympathetic dystrophy.

Postoperative radiographs should be used to verify satisfactory position of the hardware and for evidence of fracture healing. Initial radiographs are obtained immediately postoperatively, at 2 weeks, 6 weeks, and 3 months. Radiographic evidence of fracture healing will usually not become apparent until between 6 weeks and 3 months postoperatively. Resisted exercises are begun when fracture healing is apparent, usually between 6 and 8 weeks postoperatively. An early supervised rehabilitation program is critical to the success of fracture fixation, as a stiff shoulder, elbow, or hand may severely compromise the operative result.

REFERENCES

1. Henry AK. Extensile Exposure. 2d ed. Baltimore: The Williams and Wilkins Company, 1957.
2. Bourne MH, Wood MB, Carmichael SW. Locating the lateral antebrachial cutaneous nerve. J Hand Surg 1987; 12A:697–699.
3. Siegel DB, Gelberman RH. Radial nerve: applied anatomy and operative exposure. In: Gelberman RH. Operative Nerve Repair and Reconstruction. Philadelphia: Lippincott, 1991:393–407.
4. Hoppenfeld S, deBoer P. Surgical Exposures in Orthopaedics: The Anatomic Approach. 2d ed. Philadelphia: J.B. Lippincott Company, 1994.
5. Ulrich C. Surgical treatment of humeral diaphyseal fractures. In: Flatow EL, Ulrich C. Humerus. Oxford: Butterworth-Heinemann, 1996:128–143.
6. Bauer R, Kerschbaumer F, Poisel S. Operative Approaches in Orthopedic Surgery and Traumatology. New York: Thieme Medical Publishers, 1987.
7. Siegel DB, Gelberman RH. Ulnar nerve: applied anatomy and operative exposure. In: Gelberman RH. Operative Nerve Repair and Reconstruction. Philadelphia: Lippincott, 1991:413–424.
8. Sunderland S. Metrical and non-metrical features of the muscular branches of the radial nerve. J Comp Neurol 1946; 85:93–97.
9. Foster R, Dixon GL, Bach AW, Green TM. Internal fixation of fractures and non-unions of the humeral shaft. J Bone Joint Surg 1985; 67-A(6):857–864.
10. Bell MJ, Beauchamp CG, Kellam JK, McMurtry RY. The results of plating humeral shaft fractures in patients with multiple injuries. J Bone Joint Surg 1985; 6-B(2):293–296.
11. Dabezies EJ, Banta CJ, Murphy CP, D'Ambrosia RD. Plate fixation of the humeral shaft for acute fractures, with and without radial nerve injuries. J Orth Trauma 1992; 6(1):10–13.
12. Vandergriend R, Tomasin J, Ward EF. Open reduction and internal fixation of humeral shaft fractures, results using AO plating techniques. J Bone Joint Surg 1986; 68-A(3):430–433.
13. Chapman JR, Henley MB, Agel J, et al. Randomized prospective study of humeral shaft fracture fixation: intramedullary nails versus plates. J Orthop Trauma 2000; 14:162–166.
14. McCormack RG, Brien BD, Buckley RE, et al. Fixation of fractures of the shaft of the humerus by dynamic compression plate or intramedullary nail: a prospective randomised trial. J Bone Joint Surg 2000; 82-B:336–339.
15. Ring D, Jupiter J, Quintero J, Sanders R, Marti RK. Atrophic uninited diaphyseal fractures of the humerus with a bony defect: treatment by wave plate osteosynthesis. J Bone Joint Surg 2000; 82-B(6):867–871.
16. Crates J, Whittle AP. Antegrade interlocking nailing of acute humeral shaft fractures. Clin Orthop 1998; 350:40–50.
17. Ipkme JO. Intramedullary interlocking nailing for humeral fractures: experiences with the Russell-Taylor humeral nail. Injury 1994; 25:447–455.
18. Rommens PM, Verbruggen J, Broos PL. Retrograde locked nailing of humeral shaft fractures. J Bone Joint Surg 1995; 77-B(1):84–89.
19. Rommens PM, Blum J, Runkel M. Retrograde nailing of humeral shaft fractures. Clin Orthop 1998; 350:26–39.
20. Lin J, Hou S, Hang Y, Chao E. Treatment of humeral shaft fractures by retrograde locked nailing. Clin Orthop 1997; 342:147–155.
21. Hinsenkamp M, Burny F, Andrianne Y, Quintin J, Rasquin C, Donkerwolcke M, Picchio AA, Asche G. External fixation of the fracture of the humerus: a review of 164 cases. Orthopedics 1984; 7(8):1309–1314.

22. De Bastiani G, Aldegheri R, Reni Brivio L. The treatment of fractures with a dynamic external fixator. J Bone Joint Surg 1984; 66-B:538–545.

23. Lammens J, Bauduin G, Driesen R, Moens P, Stuyck J, De Smet L, Fabry G. Treatment of non-union of the humerus using the Ilizarov external fixator. Clin Orthop 1998; 353:223–230.

24. Cattaneo R, Catagni MA, Guerreschi F. Application of the Ilizarov method in the humerus: lengthenings and non-unions. Hand Clin 1993; 9(4):729–739.

25. Ring D, Jupiter J, Toh S. Salvage of contaminated fractures of the distal humerus with thin wire external fixation. Clin Orthop 1999; 359:203–208.

26. Rosen H. The treatment of non-unions and pseudarthroses of the humeral shaft. Orth Clin North Am 1990; 21(40):725–742.

27. Jupiter J, Von Deck M. Uninited humeral diaphysis. J Shoulder Elbow Surg 1998; 7(6):644–653.

28. McKee MD, Miranda M, Riemer BL, Blasier RB, Redmond BJ, Sims SH, Waddell JP, Jupiter JB. Management of humeral non-union after the failure of locking intramedullary nails. J Orthop Trauma 1996; 10(7):492–499.

29. Jupiter J. Complex non-union of the humeral diaphysis: treatment with a medial approach, an anterior plate, and a vascularized fibular graft. J Bone Joint Surg 1990; 72-A(5):701–707.

Index